C. M. Wormington, Ph.D., O.D.

Neuro-Ophthalmology

Review Manual

Fifth Edition

Neuro-Ophthalmology

Review Manual

Fifth Edition

Lanning B. Kline, MD

Frank J. Bajandas, MD

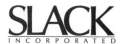

SLACK
INCORPORATED

6900 Grove Road • Thorofare, NJ 08086
an innovative information, education, and management company

Publisher: John H. Bond
Editorial Director: Amy E. Drummond
Senior Associate Editor: Jennifer Stewart

Kline, Lanning B.
    Neuro-ophthalmology review manual / Lanning B. Kline, Frank J. Bajandas.--5th ed.
        p. ; cm.
    Includes bibliographical references and index.
    ISBN 1-55642-470-1 (alk. paper)
        1. Neuro-ophthalmology--Examinations, questions, etc. I. Bajandas, Frank J. II. Title.
        [DNLM: 1. Eye Diseases--Handbooks. 2. Eye--innervation--Handbooks. 3. Eye Manifestations
        --Handbooks. 4. Neurologic Manifestations--Handbooks. WW 39 K65n 2000]
    RE725 .K55 2000
    617.7--dc21   00-057413

Printed in the United States.

Published by: SLACK Incorporated
                              6900 Grove Road
                              Thorofare, NJ 08086 USA
                              Telephone: 856-848-1000
                              Fax: 856-853-5991
                              www.slackbooks.com

Last digit is print number: 10 9 8 7 6 5 4 3 2 1

DEDICATION

Gentler the Path with Familiar Footsteps to Follow

This manual is dedicated to
Robert B. Daroff, MD
Joel S. Glaser, MD
J. Lawton Smith, MD

CONTENTS

About the Authors

Lanning B. Kline, MD
Alabama Eye Institute Professor and
Chairman, Department of Ophthalmology
University of Alabama School of Medicine
Birmingham, Alabama

Frank J. Bajandas, MD
Associate Clinical Professor
Department of Ophthalmology
University of Texas Health Science Center
San Antonio, Texas
Deceased

Contributing Authors

Richard H. Fish, MD
Vitreo-Retinal Consultants
Clinical Associate Professor
Department of Ophthalmology
Baylor College of Medicine
Houston, Texas

Christopher A. Girkin, MD
Assistant Professor
Department of Ophthalmology
University of Alabama School of Medicine
Birmingham, Alabama

Saunders L. Hupp, MD
Professor of Ophthalmology and Neurology
University of South Alabama
Mobile, Alabama

Angela R. Lewis, MD
Assistant Clinical Professor
Department of Ophthalmology
University of Alabama School of Medicine
Birmingham, Alabama

Patrick S. O'Connor, MD
Clinical Professor of Ophthalmology
Department of Ophthalmology
University of Texas Health Science Center
San Antonio, Texas

Milton F. White, Jr, MD
Retina Consultants of Alabama
Assistant Professor, Department of Ophthalmology
University of Alabama School of Medicine
Birmingham, Alabama

INTRODUCTION TO THE FIFTH EDITION

In the First Edition of *Neuro-Ophthalmology Review Manual*, Frank Bajandas, MD, described the text as a "readable compendium of 'no-nonsense' neuro-ophthalmology." I have held fast to this charge in creating the Fifth Edition.

Chapters 2 and 3, dealing with control of eye movements and nystagmus, have once again been updated. This was greatly facilitated with the help of Robert Daroff, MD, of Cleveland, Ohio, and Lea Averbuch-Heller, MD, of Tel Aviv, Israel.

Two new chapters have been added. The phakomatoses, a group of diseases with diverse neuro-ophthalmologic manifestations, are reviewed by Angela Lewis, MD. Disturbances of higher visual function provide a puzzling challenge to the clinician. Christopher Girkin, MD, has done a wonderful job of organizing and succinctly describing these disorders.

Modest additions have been made to the chapters dealing with visual fields, optic atrophy, and eyelid disorders. Tables and references have been updated. Michelle McKnight once again retyped the entire manuscript (she is almost a neuro-ophthalmologist!), and David Fisher created illustrative material.

My family remains steadfast in their support, and their love energizes my life.

Enjoy the Fifth Edition of *Neuro-Ophthalmology Review Manual*. I hope it adds to your knowledge of neuro-ophthalmology, helps in preparation for OKAP and Board examinations, and, most importantly, helps you care for your patients.

LBK

Introduction to the Fourth Edition

It has been 7 years since *Neuro-Ophthalmology Review Manual* was revised. A great portion of the text only had to be updated and references made more current.

Significant alterations were made in Chapters 2 and 3, dealing with the control of eye movements and nystagmus. My thanks to Robert Daroff, MD, and Lea Averbuch-Heller, MD, who reviewed this material.

Two new chapters have been added to the Fourth Edition. Dr. Saunders Hupp has provided a review of disorders of eyelids, while Dr. Milton White has summarized the important relationship of carotid artery disease and the eye.

My thanks to Michelle McKnight, who typed the new manuscript. David Fisher both revised and created the illustrative material for the manual. A set of color plates depicting classic fortification scotomata of migraine is included. Printed on a perforated page, it can be used by the clinician in discussing migrainous visual phenomena with the patient.

The time to prepare this Fourth Edition of *Neuro-Ophthalmology Review Manual* was "stolen" from my family. I thank them for their patience, love, and understanding.

I hope the reader enjoys this manual as much as I enjoyed preparing it. Its purpose remains unchanged: to serve as a succinct text and user-friendly reference in clinical neuro-ophthalmology.

LBK

Introduction to the Third Edition

Functional or nonorganic eye disease is clearly within the realm of neuro-ophthalmology. Therefore, a chapter entitled "Hysteria and Malingering" has been added to this review manual. Dr. R.H. Fish provided this material, and the illustrations were done by David Fisher. Alterations in Figures 4-7, 6-1, and 6-3 were made, as well as minor revisions in the text. The intent of this Third Edition remains the same as the first two: to provide a handy, organized guide to the "nuts and bolts" of neuro-ophthalmology.

LBK

INTRODUCTION TO THE SECOND EDITION

Frank Bajandas' great abilities as a teacher were clearly demonstrated in the First Edition of *Neuro-Ophthalmology Board Review Manual*. He was able to organize, synthesize, and communicate the core subject material of neuro-ophthalmology in 11 chapters comprising 141 pages. While initially intended as a study guide for residents and practitioners preparing for the Boards, this manual has become widely used by residents and fellows at all levels of training, as well as a handy reference for busy clinicians.

The revision of this teaching manual was done to update and modestly expand the material covered. The concise style and schematic illustrations have been retained. Because of the widened appeal of this book, "Board" has been deleted from the title.

My thanks go to Dr. P.S. O'Connor, who contributed two chapters and critically reviewed many others. Amy Collins both revised and created many illustrations. Kathy Fleck typed the manuscript.

My family deserves special mention. Ricki, Aaron, and Evie helped me tremendously with two contributions: love and support. Finally, I must thank Frank Bajandas, who died tragically in an automobile accident. He laid the groundwork upon which to revise and expand. I hope he would be pleased with my efforts.

LBK

INTRODUCTION TO THE FIRST EDITION

This manual was to simply be a handy, readable compendium of the "no-nonsense" neuro-ophthalmology that neurologists, neurosurgeons, and ophthalmologists need in the ritual of preparing for Board exams. The good news is that the same material represents the clinical principles used in my everyday neuro-ophthalmology practice.

The bulk of the "brute-memory" material can be boiled down to eight diagrams.* If you can reproduce these eight diagrams and, in turn, recall the significance of their components, you will be readily reminded of the organization of each theme and of the anatomico-physiological and pathological concepts that form the basis of clinical neuro-ophthalmology.

FB

*Figures 1-4, 1-6, 2-10, 2-11, 3-7, 3-8, 4-3, and 9-1 (please note these figures are from the First Edition and not the Fifth Edition).

Chapter 1

Visual Fields

I. **Traquair's definition of the visual field**

   A. Island of vision in a sea of blindness (Figure 1-1). The peak of the island represents the point of highest acuity—the fovea—while the "bottomless pit" represents the blind spot—the optic disc

II. **Visual field testing**

   A. Stimuli: testing the island of vision at various levels requires targets that vary in:
       1. Size
       2. Intensity
       3. Color

   B. Field testing methods (Figure 1-2)
       1. Kinetic: mapping the contours of the island at different levels, resulting in one isopter for each level tested
       2. Static: vertical contours of the island along a selected meridian

III. **For clinical testing, the visual field can be divided into two areas (Figure 1-3)**

   A. Central: 30-degree radius

   B. Peripheral: beyond 30 degrees

IV. **Central visual field**

   A. Can be examined with an Amsler grid, confrontation techniques, tangent screen, and bowl perimeter

   B. Confrontation techniques: see Chapter 20

   C. Amsler grid—useful in detecting subtle, central, and paracentral scotomas. When held at one-third of a meter from the patient, each square subtends 1 degree of visual field

   D. Tangent screen (campimetry) is an excellent method to examine the central field. Easier to pick up central defects with tangent screen versus bowl perimeter. Scotomas will be three times as large at 1 meter with tangent screen as on the perimeter test surface, which is only one-third meter from the patient

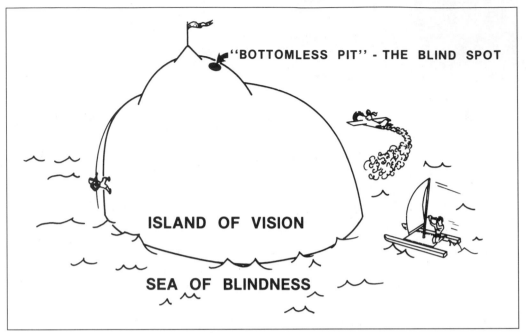

Figure 1-1. Traquair's definition of the visual field—island of vision in a sea of blindness.

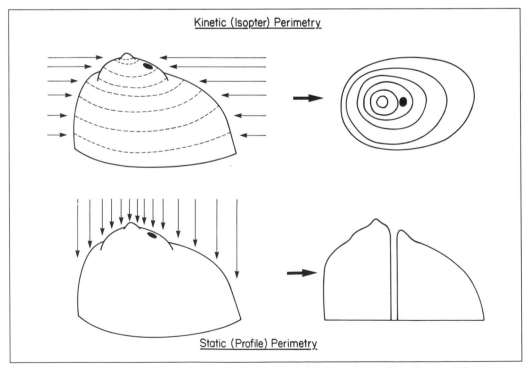

Figure 1-2. Kinetic perimetry: each set of target size-color-intensity and background illumination determines a different level of the island being tested and results in a different oval-shaped cross-section or isopter; note the six isopters at the right, the result of testing six levels of the island. Static perimetry: the target is held stationary at different points along the selected meridians; the intensity of the target is slowly increased until it is detected by the patient; the intensity required determines the upper level (the greatest sensitivity) of the island at this point.

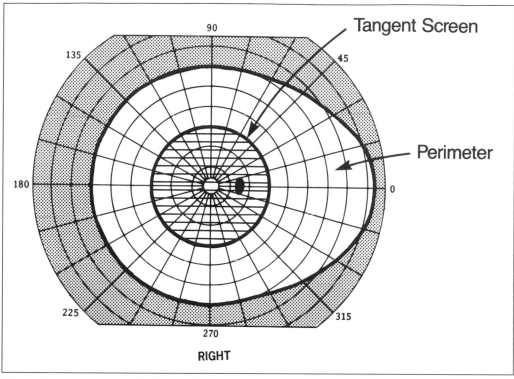

Figure 1-3. Central visual field (30-degree radius) can be tested with a tangent screen, while the entire field can be tested with a perimeter.

    E. Tangent screen not useful for testing beyond 30 degrees because of diminishing stimulus value of test object on flat testing surface; bowl perimeter (eg, manual, automated) can also be used to test central 30 degrees

V.   Peripheral visual field

    A. Requires testing with bowl perimeter

    B. Automated perimetry able to examine central 60 degrees

    C. Manual perimetry tests entire visual field

    D. Particularly helpful in detecting:
        1. Ring scotoma (retinitis pigmentosa)
        2. Nasal step (glaucoma)
        3. Temporal crescent (occipital lobe)

VI. Anatomy of the visual pathways (Figure 1-4)

    A. The visual field and retina have an inverted and reversed relationship. Relative to the point of fixation, the upper visual field falls on the inferior retina (below the fovea), lower visual field on the superior retina, nasal visual field on the temporal retina, and temporal visual field on the nasal retina

    B. Nasal fibers of ipsilateral eye cross in the chiasm join uncrossed temporal fibers of the contralateral eye → optic tract → synapse in lateral geniculate nucleus → optic radiation → terminate in the visual cortex (area 17) of the occipital lobe

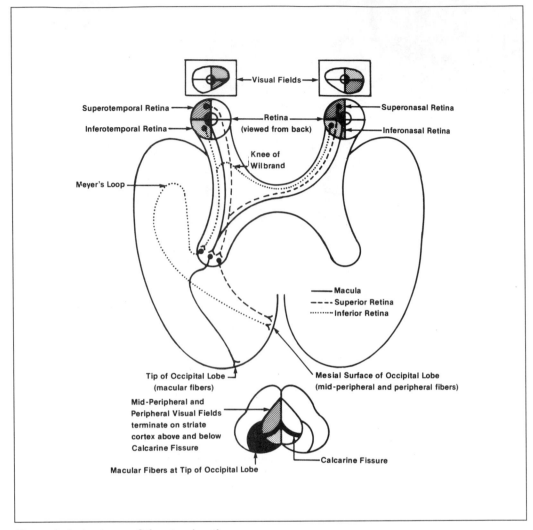

Figure 1-4. Anatomy of the visual pathways.

C. Inferonasal retinal fibers decussate in the chiasm and travel anteriorly in the contralateral optic nerve before passing into the optic tract. They form "Wilbrand's knee"

D. While the presence of Wilbrand's knee has been challenged (Horton, 1997), it still appears to have clinical relevance (Karanjia and Jacobson, 1999)

E. Lower retinal fibers and their projections lie in the lateral portion of the optic tract and ultimately terminate in the inferior striate cortex on the lower bank of the calcarine fissure. Upper retinal fibers project through the medial optic tract and ultimately terminate in the superior striate cortex

F. The central (30 degrees) visual field occupies a disproportionately large area (83%) of the visual cortex. The vertical hemianopic meridians are represented along the border of the calcarine lips, while the horizontal meridian follows the contour of the base of the calcarine fissure (Figure 1-5)

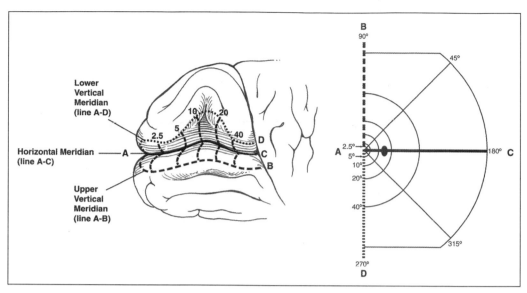

Figure 1-5. Medial view of the left occipital lobe with calcarine fissure opened, exposing the striate cortex. Dashed and solid lines represent coordinates of the visual field.

VII. Interpretation of visual field defects

A. Ten key points to remember

    1. Optic nerve-type field defects

    2. "Rules of the road" for the optic chiasm

    3. Optic tract—lateral geniculate nucleus (LGN) defects

    4. Superior-inferior separation in the temporal lobe

    5. Superior-inferior separation in the parietal lobe

    6. Central homonymous hemianopia

    7. Macular sparing

    8. Congruity

    9. Optokinetic nystagmus (OKN)

    10. Temporal crescents

B. Optic nerve-type field defects

    1. Retinal nerve fibers enter the optic discs in a specific manner (Figure 1-6)

    2. Nerve fiber bundle (NFB) defects are of the following three main types:

        a. Papillomacular bundle: macular fibers that enter the temporal aspect of the disc. A defect in this bundle of nerve fibers results in one of the following:

            i. Central scotoma (Figure 1-7): a defect covering central fixation

            ii. Centrocecal scotoma (see Figure 1-7): a central scotoma connected to the blind spot (cecum)

            iii. Paracentral scotoma (see Figure 1-7): a defect of some of the fibers of the papillomacular bundle lying next to, but not involving, central fixation

        b. Arcuate nerve fiber bundle: fibers from the retina temporal to the disc enter the superior and inferior poles of the disc (see Figure 1-6). A defect of these bundles may cause one of the following:

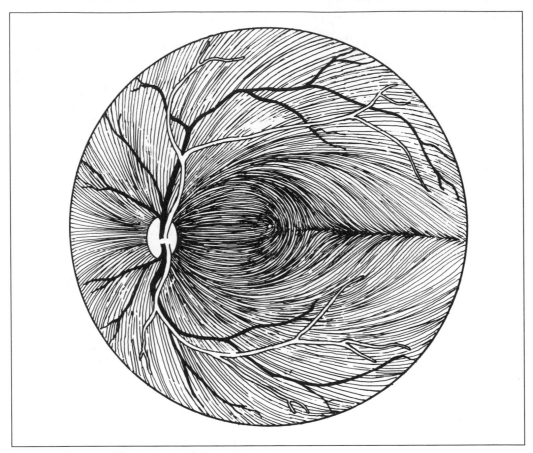

Figure 1-6. Nerve fiber pattern of the retina.

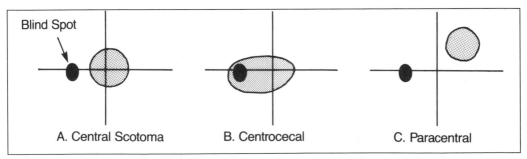

Figure 1-7. Field defects due to interruption of the papillomacular bundle.

    i. Bjerrum, arcuate, or "scimitar" scotoma (Figure 1-8): this arcuate portion of the field, at 15 degrees from fixation, is known as "Bjerrum's area"

    ii. Seidel scotoma (see Figure 1-8): a defect in the proximal portion of the NFB, causing a comma-shaped extension of the blind spot

    iii. Nasal step (of Rönne) (see Figure 1-8): a defect in the distal portion of the arcuate NFB. Since the superior and inferior arcuate bundles do not

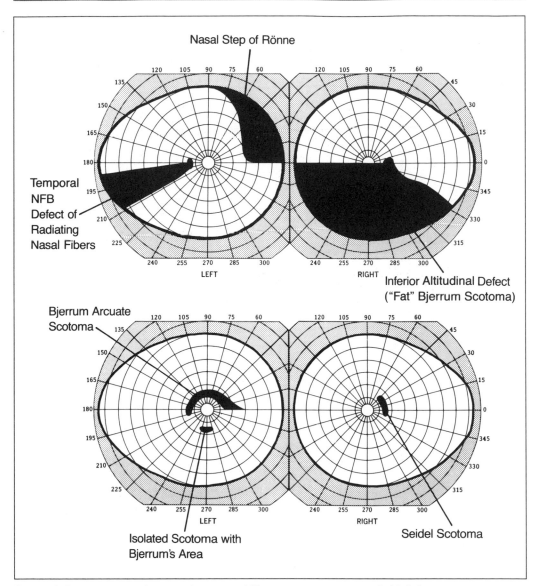

Figure 1-8. Composite diagram depicting different optic nerve-type field defects.

cross the horizontal raphe of the temporal retina, a nasal step defect respects the horizontal (180 degrees) meridian

    iv. Isolated scotoma within Bjerrum's area (see Figure 1-8): defect of the intermediate portion of the arcuate NFB

  c. Nasal nerve fiber bundles: fibers that enter the nasal aspect of the disc course in a straight (nonarcuate) fashion. The defect in this bundle results in a wedge-shaped temporal scotoma arising from the blind spot and does not necessarily respect the temporal horizontal meridian (see Figure 1-8)

3. Lesions at or behind the chiasm tend to cause hemianopic field defects originating from the point of fixation and respecting the vertical meridian

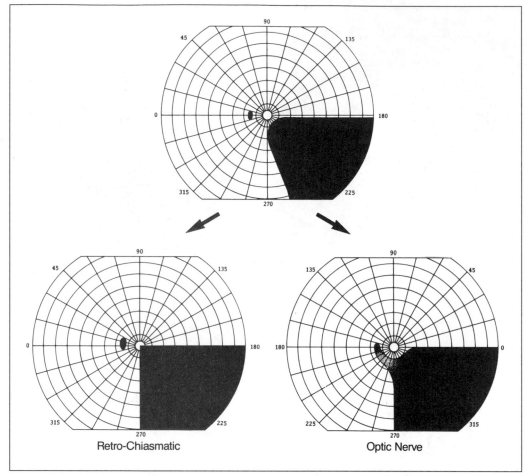

Figure 1-9. The key question in a patient with a quadrantic visual field defect: Does the field defect go to fixation (retrochiasmatic lesion) or to the blind spot (optic nerve lesion)?

4. Optic nerve lesions cause field defects corresponding to one of the three major NFB defects described above. Nerve fiber bundle defects originate from the blind spot, not from the fixation point, and do not respect the vertical meridian, but do respect the nasal horizontal meridian

5 The key question, therefore, in a patient with a quadrantic field defect is: does the field defect go to fixation or to the blind spot (Figure 1-9)?

6. Additional clinical findings supporting the diagnosis of optic neuropathy as the cause of the field defect include:

    a. Decreased visual acuity: patients with isolated retrochiasmatic lesions do not have decreased visual acuity unless the lesions are bilateral, then the visual acuities will be equal; if a patient has hemianopic field defects with unequal visual acuities, then look for a lesion around the chiasm (affecting the optic nerves asymmetrically)

    b. Patients with decreased (or suspected decreased) visual acuity can be further tested with:

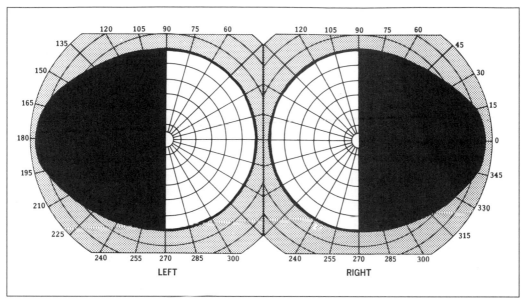

Figure 1-10. Bitemporal hemianopia due to interruption of decussating nasal fibers in the chiasm.

   i. Light-brightness comparison (eye with optic neuropathy will see the light as "less bright")

   ii. Color perception comparison (color plates or Mydriacyl bottle cap) (eye with optic neuropathy will have diminished color perception)

   iii. Light-stress recovery time (eye with maculopathy will have delayed recovery visual acuity after bleaching with light)

   iv. Afferent pupillary defect test ("swinging flashlight" or Marcus Gunn test—see Chapter 8)

   v. Tests i through iv may help in distinguishing cases of decreased visual acuity due to macular disease from those due to optic nerve disease

   vi. Visually evoked potential (VEP)

   vii. Ophthalmoscopic evidence of optic disc abnormality (eg, pallor, cupping, drusen)

 C. "Rules of the road" for the optic chiasm:

  1. Three rules describe the course of major fiber bundles in the chiasm:

   a. The nasal retinal fibers (including the nasal half of the macula) of each eye cross in the chiasm to the contralateral optic tract. Temporal fibers remain uncrossed. Thus, a chiasmal lesion will cause a bitemporal hemianopia due to interruption of decussating nasal fibers (Figure 1-10)

   b. Lower retinal fibers project through the optic nerve and chiasm to lie laterally in the tracts; upper retinal fibers will lie medially (there is a 90-degree rotation of fibers from the nerves through the chiasm into the tracts)

   c. Inferonasal retinal fibers cross into the chiasm and cross anteriorly approximately 4 mm in the contralateral optic nerve (Wilbrand's knee) before turning back to join uncrossed inferotemporal temporal fibers in the optic tract (junctional scotoma)

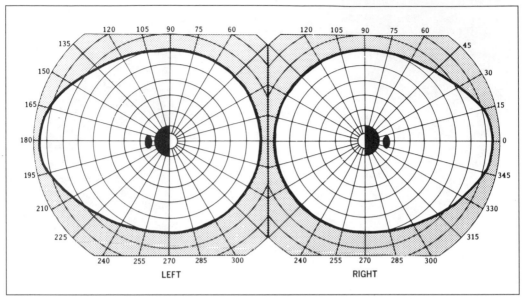

Figure 1-11. A chiasmatic lesion may affect only the decussating nasal-macular fibers, resulting in a central bitemporal hemianopia. Therefore, a complete visual field evaluation of a patient suspected of a chiasmatic lesion must include a search of the central field.

2. "Macular" crossing fibers are distributed throughout the chiasm and if primarily affected, cause a "central" bitemporal hemianopia (Figure 1-11)
3. J. Lawton Smith, MD's "super gem": if a patient comes in with poor vision in the left eye, the important eye for visual examination is the right due to involvement of Wilbrand's knee. The lesion is now intracranial at the junction of the left optic nerve and chiasm. The field defects constitute a junctional scotoma (Figure 1-12)

D. Optic tract—lateral geniculate nucleus defects
   1. All retrochiasmatic lesions result in a contralateral homonymous hemianopia
   2. Congruity describes incomplete homonymous hemianopic defects that are identical in all attributes: location, shape, size, depth, slope of margins
   3. **Remember:** the more posterior (toward the occipital cortex) the lesion in the postchiasmal visual pathways, the more likely the defects will be congruous
   4. In the optic tracts and lateral geniculate nuclei, nerve fibers of corresponding points (retinal positions of the two eyes that image the same position in visual space) do not yet lie adjacent to one another. This leads to incongruous visual field defects (Figure 1-13)
   5. Criteria for optic tract syndrome
      a. Incongruous homonymous hemianopia
      b. Bilateral retinal nerve fiber layer atrophy or optic (occasionally "bow-tie") atrophy (see Chapter 10, Section III, G, and Figure 10-2)
      c. Pupillary abnormalities
         i. Relative afferent defect: on side opposite the lesion (eye with temporal field loss)

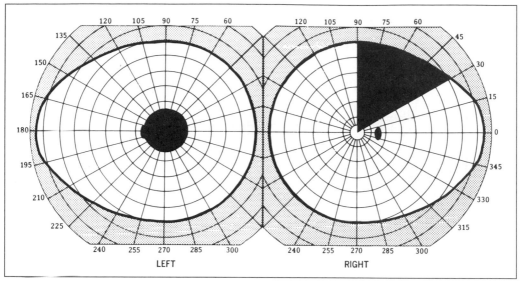

Figure 1-12. Junctional scotoma: a central scotoma in one eye with a superior-temporal defect in the fellow eye; indicates a lesion at the junction of the optic nerve (left eye in this case) and the chiasm.

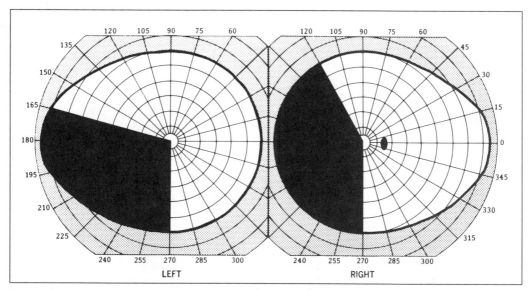

Figure 1-13. Incongruous left homonymous hemianopia due to a right optic tract lesion.

        ii. Wernicke's pupil: light stimulation of a "blind" retina causes no pupillary reaction, while light projected on an "intact" retina produces normal pupillary constriction

        iii. Behr's pupil: anisocoria with larger pupil on the side of hemianopia; probably does not exist

    6. Lateral geniculate nucleus (LGN) field defect

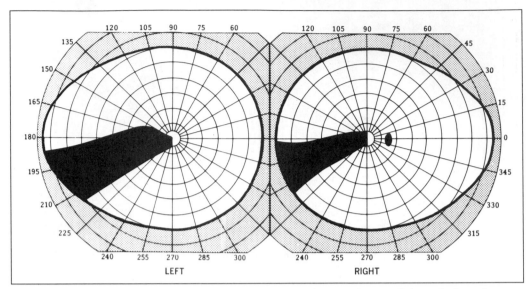

Figure 1-14. Left homonymous horizontal sectoranopia due to a lesion of the right lateral geniculate nucleus.

       a. Extremely rare

       b. Types of defects:

           i. Incongruous homonymous hemianopia

          ii. Relatively congruous homonymous horizontal sectoranopia (Figure 1-14): associated with sectorial optic atrophy; may be due to vascular infarction of a portion of the lateral geniculate body

         iii. With bilateral LGN involvement may develop hourglass-shaped visual field defects (anterior choroidal artery supplies the ventral nucleus) or hourglass-preserved defects (lateral choroidal artery supplies the dorsal nucleus)

   E. Superior-inferior separation in the temporal lobe

      1. Inferior fibers (ipsilateral inferotemporal fibers and contralateral inferonasal fibers) course anteriorly from the lateral geniculate body into the temporal lobe, forming Meyer's loop approximately 2.5 cm from the anterior tip of the temporal lobe. They are anatomically separated from the superior retinal fibers, which course directly back in the optic radiations of the parietal lobe (see Figure 1-4)

      2. Inferior "macular" fibers do not cross as far anteriorly in the temporal lobe

      3. Anterior temporal lobe lesions tend to produce midperipheral and peripheral contralateral homonymous superior quadrantanopia ("pie in the sky" field defect) (Figure 1-15)

      4. More extensive temporal lobe lesions may cause field defects that extend to the inferior quadrants, but hemianopia will be "denser" superiorly

   F. Superior-inferior separation in the parietal lobe

      1. Superior fibers (ipsilateral superotemporal fibers and contralateral superonasal fibers) course directly through the parietal lobe to lie superiorly in the optic radiation

      2. Inferior fibers course through the temporal lobe (Meyer's loop) and lie inferiorly in the optic radiation

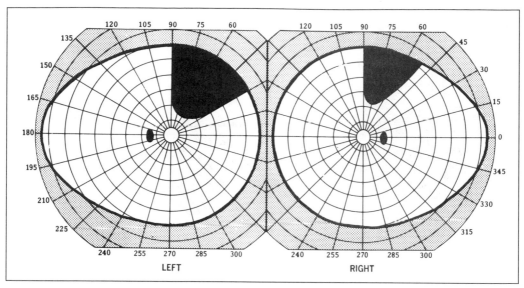

Figure 1-15. Anterior temporal lobe lesion of Meyer's loop produces incongruous, midperipheral and peripheral-contralateral, homonymous, superior ("pie in the sky") quadrantanopia. This is an example of a patient with a left temporal lobe lesion.

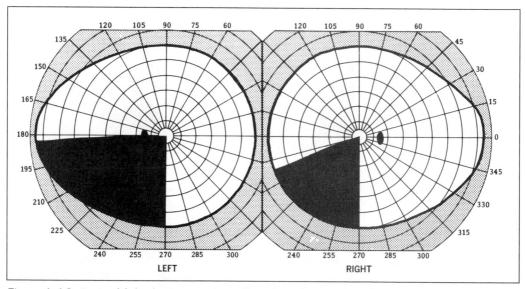

Figure 1-16. Parietal lobe lesions tend to affect the inferior, contralateral visual field quadrants first. This is an example of a patient with a right parietal lobe lesion.

3. Thus, there is "correction" of the 90-degree rotation of the visual fibers that occur through the chiasm into the tracts
4. Parietal lobe lesions tend to affect superior fibers first, resulting in contralateral inferior homonymous quadrantanopia (Figure 1-16) or a homonymous hemianopia "denser" inferiorly (Figure 1-17)

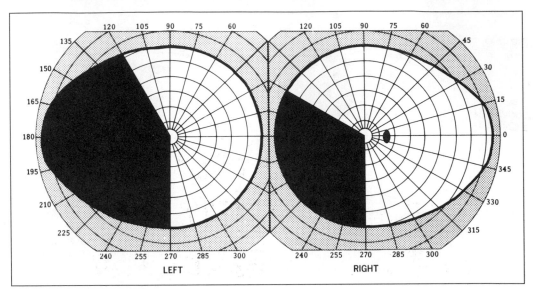

Figure 1-17. Incongruous left homonymous hemianopia.

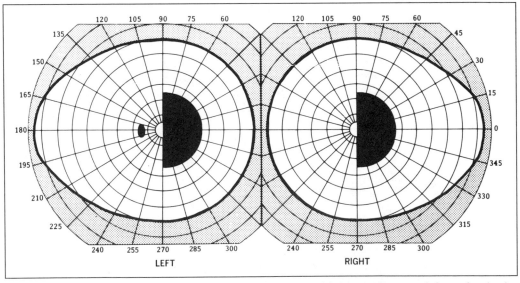

Figure 1-18. A lesion affecting only the tip of the occipital lobe produces a defect of only the central homonymous hemifields. This is an example of a patient with a left occipital tip lesion.

    5. Two signs described with parietal lobe lesions:
        a. Spasticity of conjugate gaze: tonic deviation of eyes to the side opposite a parietal lesion during an attempt to produce Bell's phenomenon (see Chapter 2)
        b. Optokinetic nystagmus asymmetry: evoked nystagmus is dampened when stimuli are moved in the direction of the damaged parietal lobe (see Section J, below)

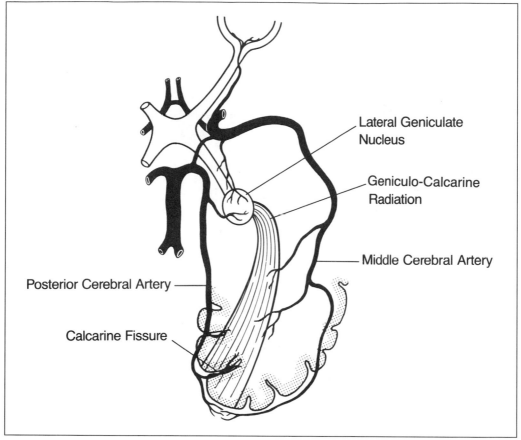

Figure 1-19. The tip of the occipital lobe, where the macular or central homonymous hemifields are represented (see Figure 1-4), is supplied by terminal branches of the middle and posterior cerebral arteries; it is referred to as a watershed area. The mesial surface of the occipital lobe is supplied by more proximal (not terminal) branches of the posterior cerebral artery.

G. Central homonymous hemianopia
   1. In the visual cortex, the macular representation is located on the tips of the occipital lobes
   2. The macular representation is separated from the cortical representation of the mid-peripheral and peripheral visual fields. These fibers terminate on the mesial surface of the occipital lobes (see Figure 1-4)
   3. A lesion affecting the tip of the occipital lobe tends to produce a central homonymous hemianopia (Figure 1-18)

H. Macular sparing
   1. The macular area of the visual cortex is a watershed area with respect to blood supply (Figure 1-19)
      a. The "macular" visual cortex is supplied by terminal branches of posterior and middle cerebral arteries

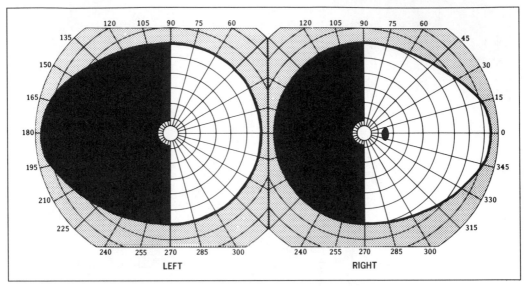

Figure 1-20. Left homonymous hemianopia with "sparing" of the left half of the macular field of each eye.

    b. The visual cortex subserving the midperipheral and peripheral field is supplied only by the posterior cerebral artery. The area is supplied by a more proximal (not a terminal) vessel

    c. Therefore, when there is obstruction of flow through the posterior cerebral artery, ipsilateral macular visual cortex may be spared because of blood supply provided by the terminal branches of the middle cerebral artery. This may be an explanation for "macular sparing"

    d. However, when there is a generalized hypoperfusion state (eg, intraoperative hypotension), the first area of the visual cortex to be affected is that supplied by terminal branches—the macular visual cortex—resulting in a central homonymous hemianopia (see Figure 1-18)

2. In order to qualify as "macular sparing," at least 5 degrees of the macular field must be spared in both eyes on the side of the hemianopia (Figure 1-20)

3. Macular sparing may at times be an artifact of testing. The patient may shift fixation, anticipating the appearance of the test object

4. If a patient with a complete homonymous hemianopia is found to have sparing of the macula, then he or she is most likely to have an occipital lobe lesion; however, the majority of patients with occipital lobe lesions demonstrate a splitting of the macula (Figure 1-21); therefore, macular sparing is helpful only if present

5. Bilateral homonymous hemianopias with macular sparing produce constricted visual fields (with normal fundi) (Figure 1-22). The differential diagnosis of constricted visual fields also includes:

    a. Hysteria/malingering

    b. Glaucoma

    c. Optic disc drusen

    d. Post-papilledema optic atrophy

    e. Retinitis pigmentosa

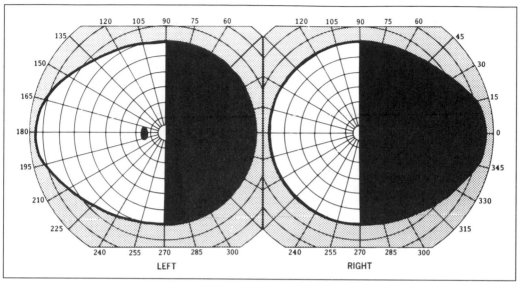

Figure 1-21. Complete right homonymous hemianopia with macular splitting.

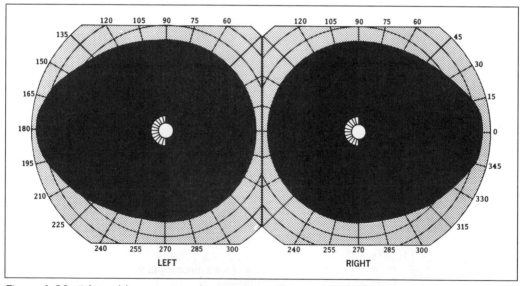

Figure 1-22. Bilateral homonymous hemianopias with macular sparing.

6. Items b through e listed above all have abnormal fundi and should be easily diagnosed. Differential from hysteria/malingering requires visual fields done at the tangent screen at 1 and 2 meters (Figure 1-23)

I. Congruity
    1. Homonymous hemianopic field defects are said to be congruous when the defect is not complete (ie, does not occupy the entire half of the field) and the defect extends to the same angular meridian in both eyes (Figure 1-24; the hemianopic defect extends to the 137-degree meridian in each eye)

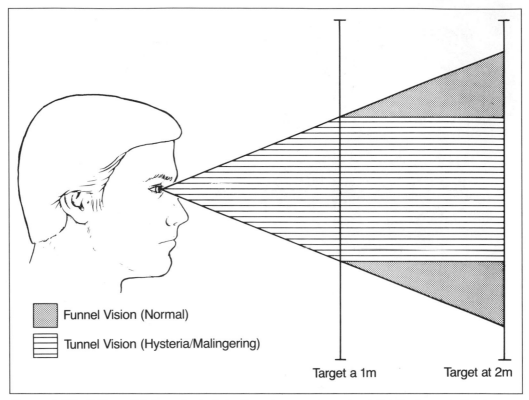

Figure 1-23. Differential from hysteria/malingering requires visual fields done at the tangent screen at 1 and 2 meters.

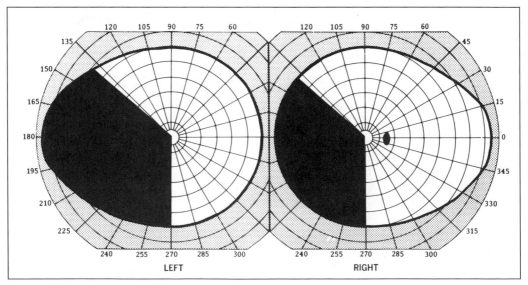

Figure 1-24. Congruous left homonymous hemianopia.

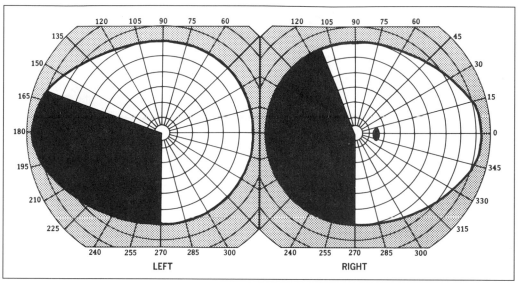

Figure 1-25. Incongruous left homonymous hemianopia.

2. Complete homonymous hemianopia (see Figure 1-21) cannot be categorized as "congruous" because it is complete

3. Figure 1-25 shows an example of incongruity: the hemianopia of the left eye extends to the 160-degree meridian while the hemianopia of the right eye extends to the 115-degree meridian

4. Optic tract lesions tend to produce markedly incongruous field defects

5. The more congruous a homonymous hemianopia, the nearer the lesion will be to the occipital cortex (ie, more posterior in the visual pathways)

6. Congruity is due to the fact that a lesion affects nerve fibers from corresponding retinal points that lie adjacent to one another

J. Optokinetic nystagmus (OKN)

1. The precise pathways of the optokinetic system are unknown in humans but may share pathways carrying smooth pursuit commands. This pathway extends from the visual association areas (18 and 19) to the horizontal gaze center in the pons (see Chapter 2)

2. The pathway in the left visual association area will terminate in the left pontine gaze center, resulting in pursuit movement of the eyes to the left. Similarly, the pathway originating in the right cerebral hemisphere generates pursuit eye movements to the right

3. A patient with a purely occipital lobe lesion (even if resulting in a complete homonymous hemianopia) will have no difficulty with pursuit, since the pathways begin more anteriorly. OKN response will be symmetric (see Figure 2-8)

4. A patient with homonymous hemianopia due to a parietal lobe lesion will have deficient pursuit eye movements to the side of the lesion, resulting in asymmetric OKN. The OKN will be decreased when the drum is rotated toward the side of the lesion (see Figure 2-9)

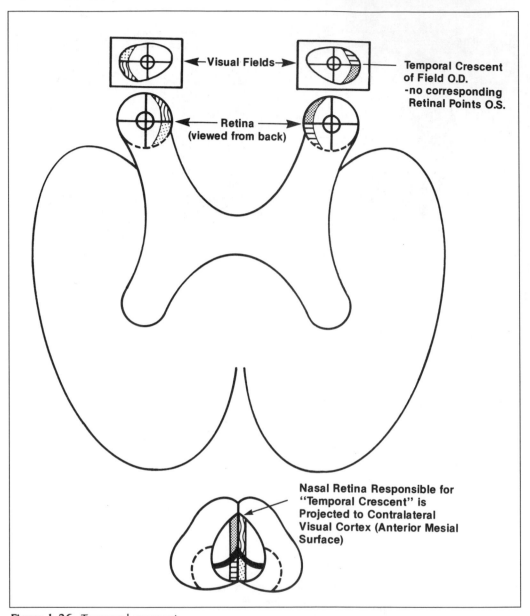

Figure 1-26. Temporal crescent.

5. Patients with homonymous hemianopia due to an optic tract, temporal lobe, or purely occipital lobe lesion will have symmetric OKN to both sides

6. Cogan's dictum

   a. Homonymous hemianopia + asymmetric OKN—probably parietal lobe lesion; most likely mass

   b. Homonymous hemianopia + symmetric OKN—probably occipital lobe lesion; most likely vascular infarction

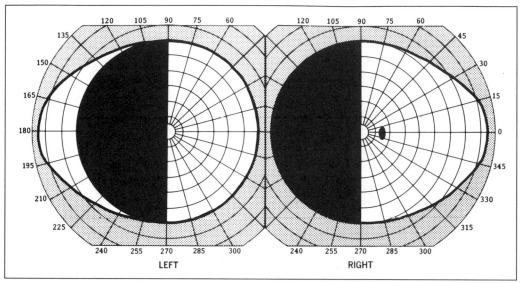

Figure 1-27. Left homonymous hemianopia with sparing of the temporal crescent of the left eye.

K. Temporal crescents
 1. When we fixate with both eyes and achieve fusion of the visual information gained by both eyes, there is superimposition of the corresponding portions of the visual fields: the central 60-degree radius of field in each eye
 2. There remains, in each eye, a temporal crescent of field for which there are no corresponding visual points in the other eye (Figure 1-26)
 3. This temporal crescent of field, perceived by a nasal crescent of retina, is represented in the contralateral visual cortex in the most anterior portion of the mesial surface of the occipital lobe (along the calcarine fissure)
 4. Representation of the temporal crescent occupies less than 10% of total surface area of striate cortex
 5. If a patient is found to have a homonymous hemianopia with sparing of the temporal crescent (Figure 1-27), then he or she probably has an occipital lobe lesion since this is the only site where the temporal crescent of fibers are separated from the other nasal fibers of the contralateral eye

VIII. Special visual field cases
A. Baring of the blind spot
 1. Baring of the blind spot in glaucoma: when a small isopter is being studied (eg, 25-degree radius, the field thus being just outside the blind spot, which is 15 to 20 degrees from fixation) the patient with Seidel scotoma (see Figure 1-8) may demonstrate a connection between the blind spot and nonseeing area outside the 25-degree radius (Figure 1-28); this is "true" baring of the blind spots
 2. A normal patient may exhibit "false" baring of the blind spot when the isopter is just outside the blind spot (see Figure 1-28)

B. Pseudobitemporal hemianopia
 1. Field defects that do not respect the vertical meridian, but rather "slope" across it (Figure 1-29)

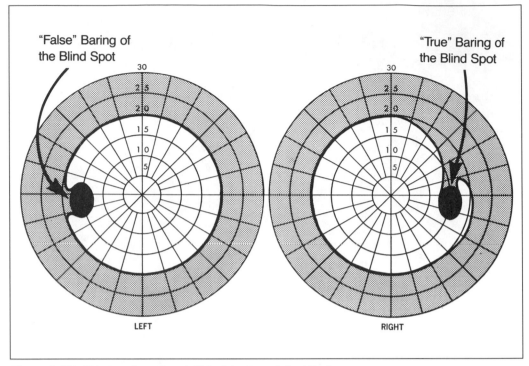

Figure 1-28. This is a "true" and "false" baring of the blind spot.

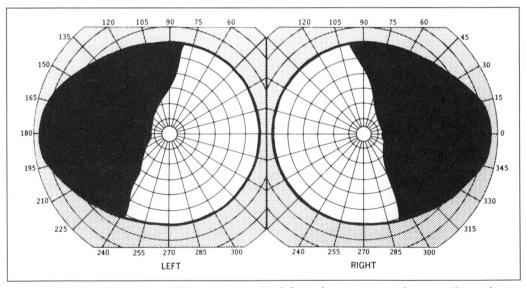

Figure 1-29. Pseudobitemporal hemianopia. Field defects do not respect the vertical meridian.

   2. Causes include:
      a. Uncorrected refractive errors (myopia, astigmatism)
      b. Tilted optic discs
      c. Enlarged blind spots in papilledema
      d. Large central or centrocecal scotomas
      e. Sectoral retinitis pigmentosa (mainly in nasal quadrants)
      f. Overhanging eyelid tissue

C. Binasal hemianopia
   1. Most nasal field defects are due to arcuate scotomas
   2. Rarely, true unilateral or bilateral nasal hemianopia may occur with defects having no arcuate connection to the blind spot and, to some extent, respecting the vertical meridian
   3. Never as a result of chiasmal compression
   4. May be due to pressure upon the temporal aspect of the optic nerve and the anterior angle of the chiasm or near the optic canal; in these locations, a lesion may affect only temporal retinal fibers. The fibers cannot be selectively obstructed in the lateral chiasm
   5. Cause includes aneurysm, tumor (pituitary adenoma), vascular infarction

VISUAL FIELD QUIZ

1. Test yourself in the interpretation of the following hypothetical cases (Figures E1 to E33).

2. Unless stated otherwise, assume that the visual fields have been evaluated with a perimeter using the same stimulus and testing conditions for each eye.

3. Describe and categorize the visual field defects and suggest the probable localization and possible causes of the lesion(s).

4. Develop a systematic approach that includes a review of the "Ten Key Points to Remember."

5. Remember the significance of altered visual acuities (see Section VII, B, 6)

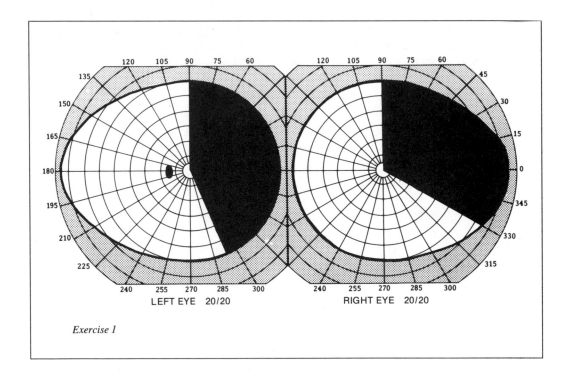

LEFT EYE   20/20   RIGHT EYE   20/20

Exercise 1

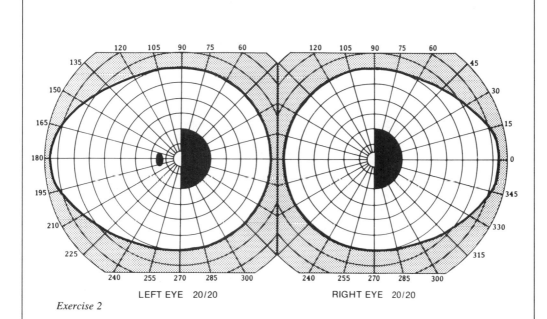

LEFT EYE   20/20   RIGHT EYE   20/20

Exercise 2

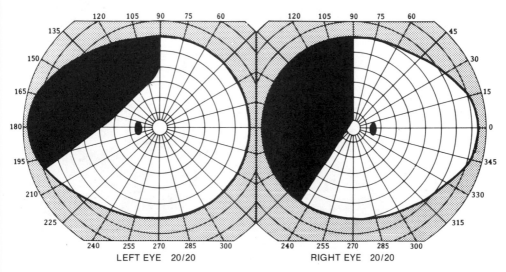

LEFT EYE   20/20   RIGHT EYE   20/20

Exercise 3

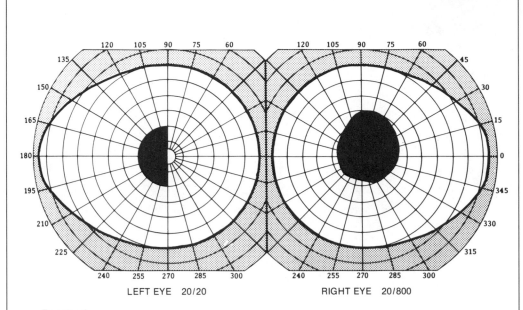

LEFT EYE   20/20

RIGHT EYE   20/800

Exercise 4

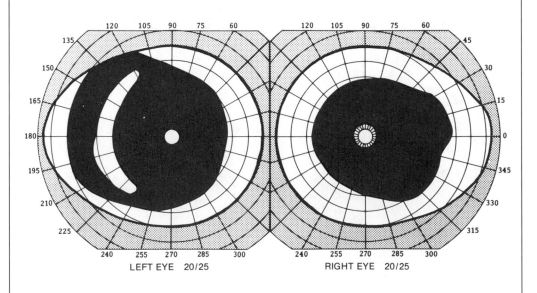

LEFT EYE   20/25

RIGHT EYE   20/25

Exercise 5

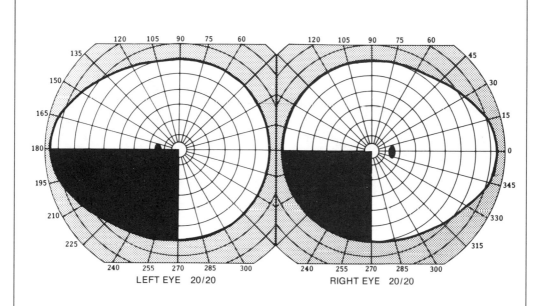

LEFT EYE   20/20   RIGHT EYE   20/20

Exercise 6

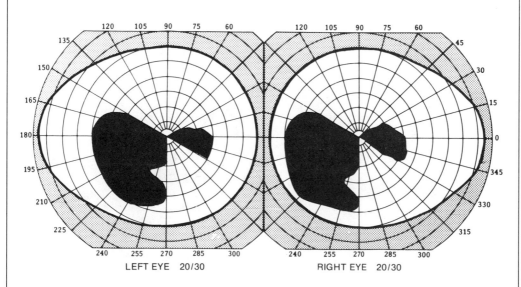

LEFT EYE   20/30   RIGHT EYE   20/30

Exercise 7

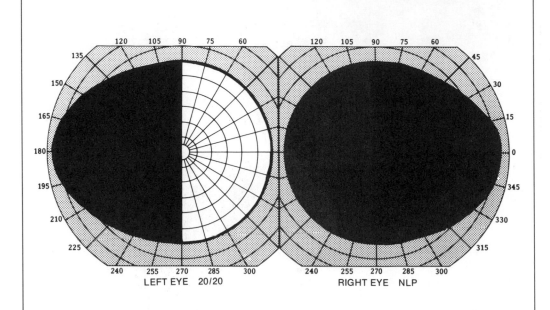

LEFT EYE 20/20   RIGHT EYE NLP

Exercise 8

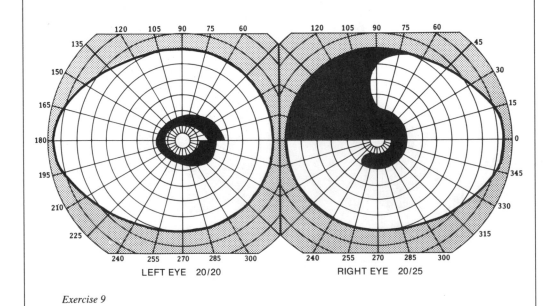

LEFT EYE 20/20   RIGHT EYE 20/25

Exercise 9

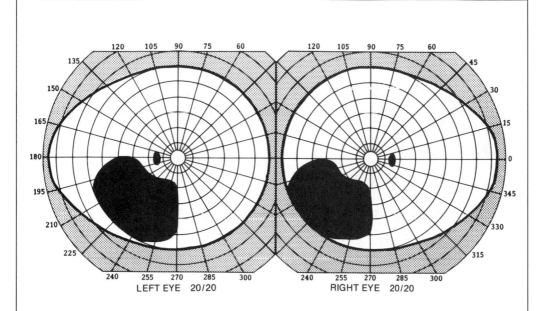

LEFT EYE 20/20   RIGHT EYE 20/20

Exercise 10

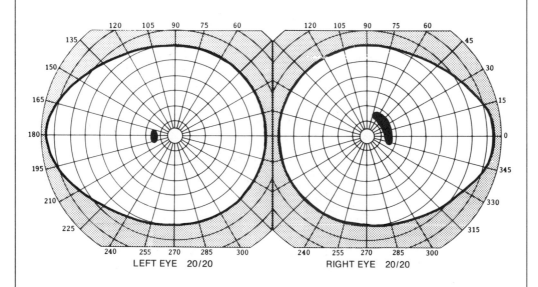

LEFT EYE 20/20   RIGHT EYE 20/20

Exercise 11

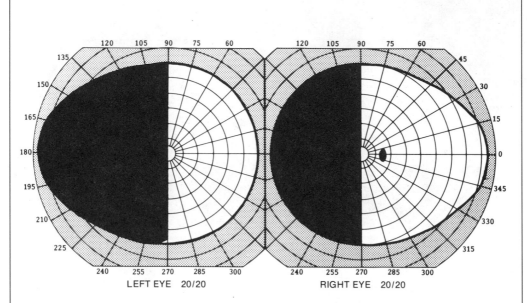

LEFT EYE 20/20   RIGHT EYE 20/20

Exercise 12

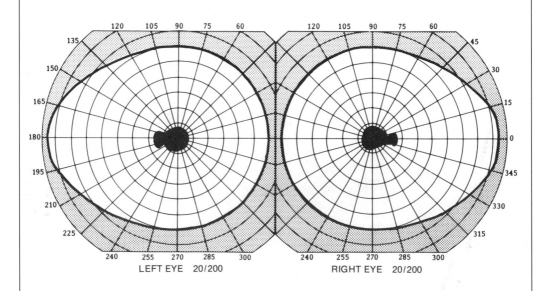

LEFT EYE 20/200   RIGHT EYE 20/200

Exercise 13

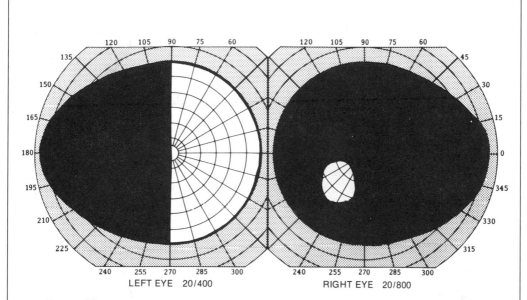

LEFT EYE   20/400   RIGHT EYE   20/800

Exercise 14

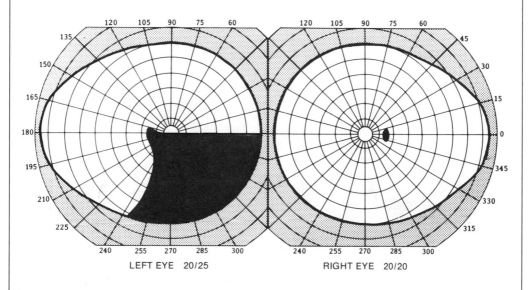

LEFT EYE   20/25   RIGHT EYE   20/20

Exercise 15

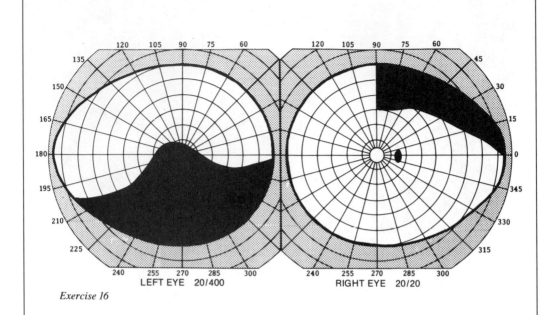

LEFT EYE   20/400   RIGHT EYE   20/20

Exercise 16

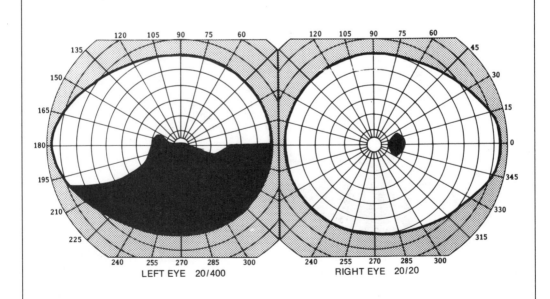

LEFT EYE   20/400   RIGHT EYE   20/20

Exercise 17

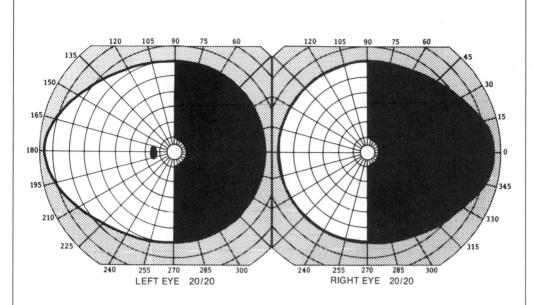

LEFT EYE   20/20   RIGHT EYE   20/20

Exercise 18

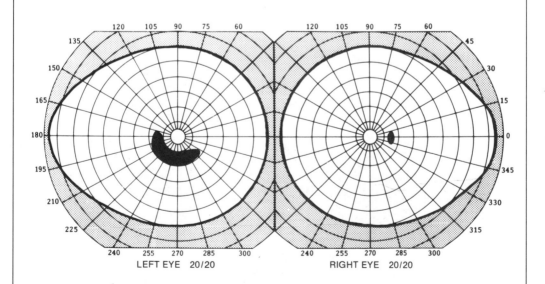

LEFT EYE   20/20   RIGHT EYE   20/20

Exercise 19

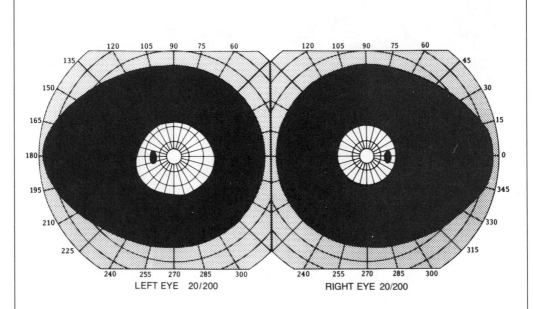

LEFT EYE 20/200   RIGHT EYE 20/200

Exercise 20-A

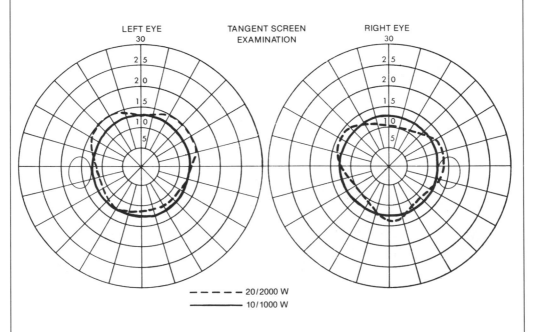

LEFT EYE   TANGENT SCREEN   RIGHT EYE
EXAMINATION

– – – – – 20/2000 W
————— 10/1000 W

Exercise 20-B

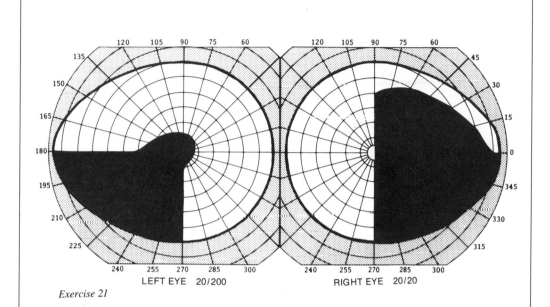

LEFT EYE   20/200   RIGHT EYE   20/20

Exercise 21

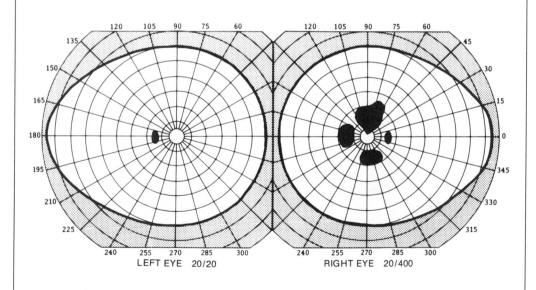

LEFT EYE   20/20   RIGHT EYE   20/400

Exercise 22

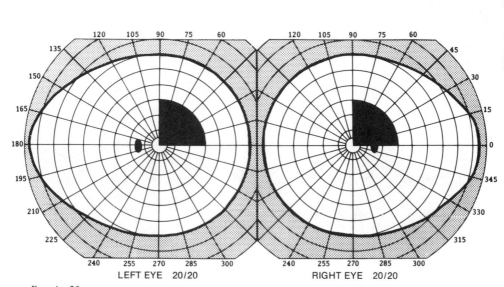

LEFT EYE   20/20

RIGHT EYE   20/20

Exercise 23

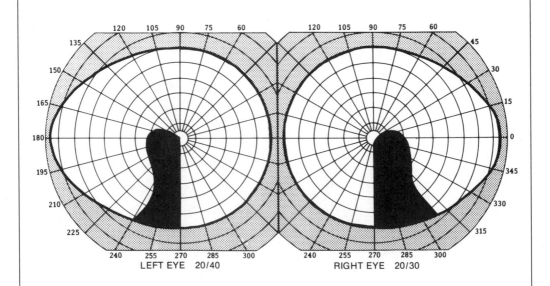

LEFT EYE   20/40

RIGHT EYE   20/30

Exercise 24

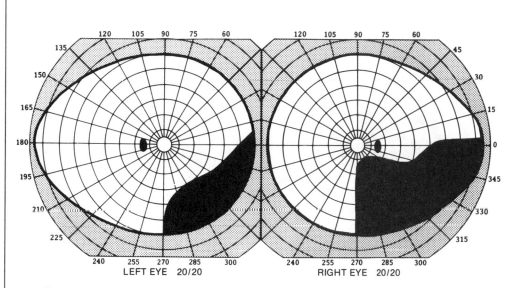

LEFT EYE   20/20

RIGHT EYE   20/20

Exercise 25

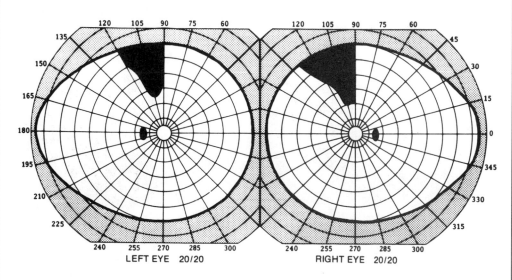

LEFT EYE   20/20

RIGHT EYE   20/20

Exercise 26

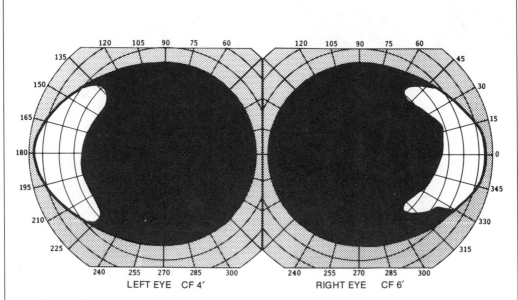

LEFT EYE   CF 4′

RIGHT EYE   CF 6′

Exercise 27

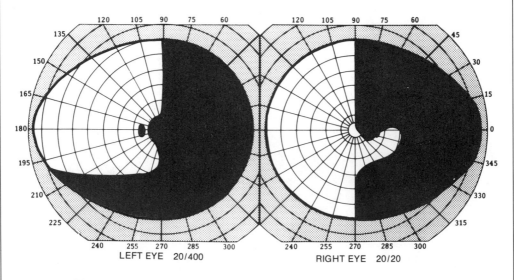

LEFT EYE   20/400

RIGHT EYE   20/20

Exercise 28

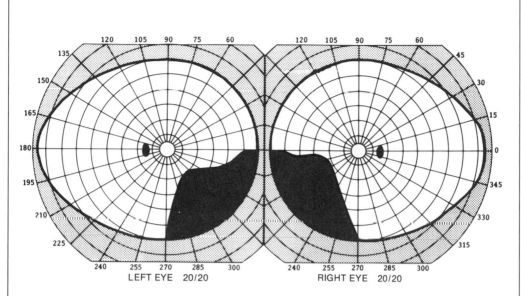

Exercise 29

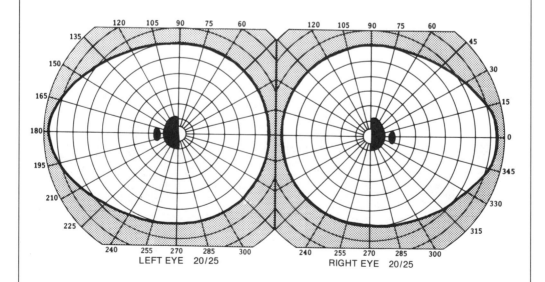

Exercise 30

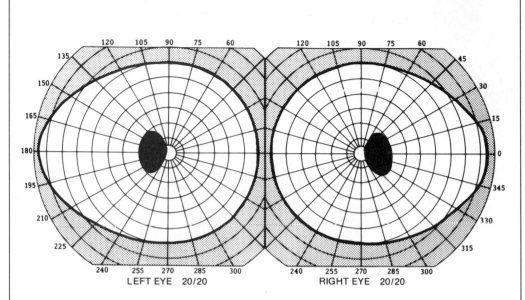

LEFT EYE   20/20

RIGHT EYE   20/20

Exercise 31

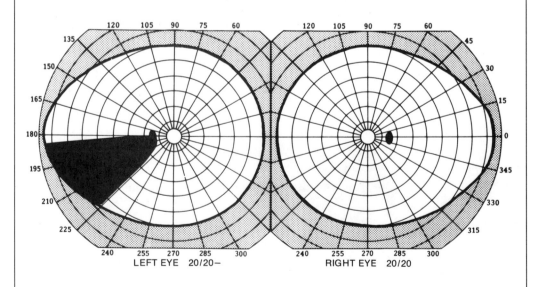

LEFT EYE   20/20−

RIGHT EYE   20/20

Exercise 32

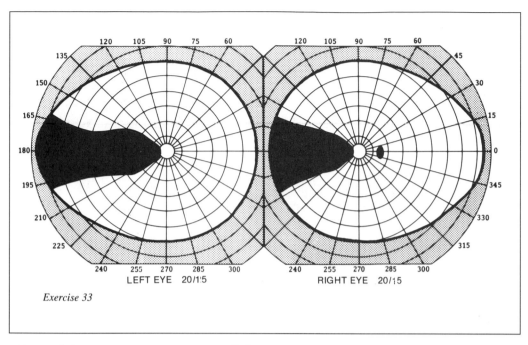

LEFT EYE 20/1'5 RIGHT EYE 20/15

Exercise 33

Plausible Interpretations of the Mystery Visual Field Defects

E1. R homonymous hemianopia, incongruous, denser above but extending to fixation and into the inferior quadrants. L temporal lobe lesion extending to the L parietal lobe.

E2. R homonymous hemianopia, central (macular), congruous. L occipital tip.

E3. L homonymous hemianopia, denser above, markedly incongruous. Marked incongruity suggests possibility of R optic tract lesion, but greater density above suggests possibility of R temporal lobe lesion, which would also be 10 times more likely statistically.

E4. R central scotoma; L central (macular) temporal hemianopia. R optic nerve lesion at the junction of the nerve and chiasm.

E5. Bilateral ring scotomas with preservation of central 10 to 20 degrees with vision of 20/25 OU. Retinitis pigmentosa versus advanced glaucoma.

E6. L homonymous inferior quadrantanopia, congruous. R parietal versus occipital lesion. The congruity gives the edge to the occipital localization.

E7. Bilateral incomplete homonymous hemianopias, congruous. Bilateral occipital lesions.

E8. Blind OD with temporal hemianopia OS. R optic nerve lesion extending into the chiasm.

E9. Double Bjerrum scotoma OS, creating a "ring" scotoma. OD: inferior arcuate scotoma (incomplete Bjerrum scotoma); superior Bjerrum scotoma breaking through nasally to create a peripheral nasal step of Rönne. Glaucoma.

E10. L homonymous inferior quadrantanopia, congruous, with sparing of temporal crescent OS, and bilateral macular sparing. R occipital lesion, upper bank of the calcarine fissure.

E11. R superior Seidel scotoma. Glaucoma. Expect to see inferior elongation of the right cup.

E12. L homonymous hemianopia, complete (cannot make statement about congruity). R optic tract, parietal, or occipital lesion. OKN asymmetry would identify the parietal cases.

E13. Bilateral centrocecal scotomas. Bilateral optic neuropathy.

E14. Inferior nasal island remaining OD. Temporal hemianopia with involvement of central field OS. Extensive chiasmatic lesion.

E15. Inferior ("fat" Bjerrum scotoma) altitudinal defect OS. OD normal. OS optic nerve lesion: glaucoma versus ischemic optic neuropathy.

E16. Inferior ("fat" Bjerrum scotoma) altitudinal defect OS with involvement of central field. Superior temporal cut OD. Lesion at junction of L optic nerve and chiasm (junctional scotoma).

E17. Inferior ("fat" Bjerrum scotoma) altitudinal defect OS with involvement of the central field. Enlarged blind spot OD. Intracranial left optic nerve lesion. We suspect that the lesion is intracranial because the right optic disc appears to be edematous, probably due to increased intracranial pressure caused by the left optic nerve tumor (meningioma). Expect to see the disc changes associated with the Foster Kennedy syndrome (optic atrophy OS and disc edema OD).

E18. R homonymous hemianopia, complete, with macular sparing. L occipital cortex.

E19. Inferior arcuate scotoma (nerve fiber bundle defect; incomplete Bjerrum scotoma) OS. OD normal. Look for disc changes. Superior elongation of the cup (glaucoma). Lumpy disc (drusen).

E20. Tubular fields with discrepancy of size of remaining fields when comparing perimeter (20-A) and tangent screen (20-B) fields. "Tunnel" vision. Functional field defects.

E21. Bitemporal hemianopia with central scotoma OS. Chiasm.

E22. Multiple central and paracentral defects OD. OS normal. Retinal lesions (chorioretinitis).

E23. R homonymous superior quadrantanopia, congruous, central, involving macular field. L occipital tip, inferior calcarine cortex.

E24. Bitemporal inferior quadrantanopia. Chiasmatic lesion with some involvement of the crossed macular fibers, causing slightly decreased acuities.

E25. R homonymous, inferior quadrantanopia, markedly incongruous. L parietal versus L optic tract.

E26. L homonymous superior quadrantanopia incongruous. "Pie in the sky" defects. R temporal lobe (Meyer's loop) lesion.

E27. Temporal islands remaining OU. Endstage glaucoma.

E28. R homonymous hemianopia, incongruous, with central scotoma OS. L optic tract lesion at junction of tract and chiasm, affecting some of the crossing macular fibers of the left eye, causing decreased acuity in that eye.

E29. Bilateral inferior nasal contraction. Optic nerve or retinal lesions (optic disc drusen, glaucoma, retinoschisis).

E30. Bitemporal hemianopia, central (macular). Chiasm.

E31. Enlarged blind spots OU, causing pseudobitemporal (central) hemianopia: papilledema.

E32. Inferior-temporal wedge-shaped field defect OS. OD normal. A nerve fiber bundle defect affecting the superior-nasal bundle of nerve fibers (see Figures 1-6, 1-8). An uncommon but well-documented glaucomatous field defect. May also represent the residual of papillitis.

E33. Congruous horizontal wedge-shaped left sectoranopia, a rare field defect due to a lesion of right lateral geniculate nucleus.

BIBLIOGRAPHY

Books

Anderson DR. *Perimetry: With and Without Automation.* 2nd ed. St. Louis, Mo: CV Mosby; 1987.

Bundez PL. *Atlas of Visual Fields.* Philadelphia, Pa: Lippincott-Raven; 1997.

Traquair HM. *Clinical Perimetry.* 7th ed. London: Henry Kimpton; 1957.

Trobe JD, Glaser JS. *The Visual Fields Manual.* Gainesville, Fla: Triad Publishing Co; 1982.

Walsh TJ, ed. Visual fields: examination and interpretation. *Ophthalmology Monographs.* Vol 3. San Francisco, Calif: American Academy of Ophthalmology; 1996.

Chapters

Glaser JS. Neuro-ophthalmology. In: Duane TD, ed. *Clinical Ophthalmology.* Vol 2. Philadelphia, Pa: Lippincott-Raven; 1992: chapters 5-7.

Hollenhorst RW, Younge BR. Ocular manifestations produced by adenomas of the pituitary gland: analysis of 1000 cases. In: Kohler DO, Ross GT, eds. *Diagnosis and Treatment of Pituitary Tumors.* Amsterdam: Excerpta Medica; 1973: 53-64.

Miller NR, Newman NJ. Topical diagnosis of lesions in the visual sensory pathway. In: Miller NR, Newman NJ, eds. *Walsh and Hoyt's Clinical Neuro-ophthalmology.* Vol 1. 5th ed. Baltimore, Md: Williams & Wilkins; 1998: 237-386.

Articles

Donahue SP, Kardon RH, Thompson HS. Hourglass-shaped visual fields as a sign of bilateral lateral geniculate myelinolysis. *Am J Ophthalmol.* 1995;119:378-379.

Frisén L. Quadruple sectoranopia and sectorial optic atrophy: a syndrome of the distal anterior choroidal artery. *J Neurol Neurosurg Psychiatry.* 1979;42:590-594.

Frisén L, Holmegeard L, Rosencrantz M. Sectorial optic atrophy and homonymous, horizontal sectoranopia: a lateral choroidal artery syndrome? *J Neurol Neurosurg Psychiatry.* 1978;41:374-380.

Greenfield DS, Siatkowski RM, Schatz NJ, Glaser JS. Bilateral lateral geniculitis associated with severe diarrhea. *Am J Ophthalmol.* 1996;122:280-281.

Horton JC. Wilbrand's knee of the primate chiasm is an artifact of monocular enucleation. *Tr Am Ophthalmol Soc.* 1997;95:579-609.

Horton JC, Hoyt WF. The representation of the visual field in human striate cortex. A revision of the classic Holmes map. *Arch Ophthalmol.* 1991;109:816-824.

Hoyt WF, Luis O. The primate chiasm: details of visual fiber organization studied by silver impregnation techniques. *Arch Ophthalmol.* 1962;68:94-106.

Hoyt WF, Tudor RC. The course of parapapillary temporal retinal axons through the anterior optic nerve. A Nanta degeneration study in the primate. *Arch Ophthalmol.* 1963;69:503-507.

Karanjia N, Jacobson DM. Compression of the prechiasmatic optic nerve produces a junctional scotoma. *Am J Ophthalmol.* 1999;128:256-258.

Salinas RF, Smith IL. Binasal hemianopia. *Surg Neurol.* 1978;10:187-194.

Savino PJ, Paris M, Schatz NJ, et al. Optic tract syndrome. *Arch Ophthalmol.* 1978;96:656-663.

Smith JL. Homonymous hemianopia: a review of one hundred cases. *Am J Ophthalmol.* 1962;54:616-623.

Smith JL, Cogan DG. Optokinetic nystagmus: a test for parietal lobe lesions. *Am J Ophthalmol.* 1959;48:187-193.

Smith TJ, Baker RS. Perimetric findings in functional disorders using automated techniques. *Ophthalmology.* 1987;94:1562-1566.

Trobe JD, Lorber ML, Schlezinger NS. Isolated homonymous hemianopias: a review of 104 cases. *Arch Ophthalmol.* 1973;89:377-381.

Van Buren JM, Baldwin M. The architecture of the optic radiation in the temporal lobe of man. *Brain.* 1958;81:15-40.

Chapter 2

Supranuclear and Internuclear Gaze Pathways

I. The eyes move in six ways, two of them fast and four of them slow

A. Fast eye movements (FEM) (velocity: 100° to 600°/second)

　　1. The larger the amplitude, the higher the velocity

　　2. Saccade (French term for "jerk movement")

　　3. Nystagmus (quick phase): a rudimentary type of saccade

B. Slow eye movements (SEM) (velocity: 5° to 50°/second)

　　1. Smooth pursuit

　　2. Optokinetic

　　3. Vestibular

　　4. Vergence

II. Functional classification of eye movements (Table 2-1)

A. FEM: saccades

　　1. Stimuli

　　　　a. Voluntary changes in direction (voluntary saccade)

　　　　b. Sudden peripheral-visual, auditory, or sensory (eg, pain) stimulus (reflexive saccade)

　　2. Visual "suppression" during saccades: even though the visual world is rapidly sweeping across the retina, there is no sense of a blurred image

B. FEM: nystagmus quick phases

　　1. Stimulus: vestibular or optokinetic stimulation would lead the eyes to extreme contraversive deviation unless prevented by corrective quick phases

　　2. Provide automatic resetting movements in the presence of spontaneous drifts of the eyes

　　3. This type of FEM is the phylogenetic forerunner of voluntary saccades

C. SEM: smooth pursuit

　　1. Stimuli

　　　　a. Motion of the image of a target across the foveal and perifoveal retina

　　　　b. Occasionally nonvisual stimuli, such as proprioception, can also generate smooth pursuit movements (eg, following one's own fingers in darkness)

Table 2-1

A FUNCTIONAL CLASSIFICATION OF HUMAN EYE MOVEMENTS

Class of Eye Movements	Main Function
Saccades	To bring objects of interest onto the fovea
Nystagmus quick phases	To reset the eyes during prolonged rotation and direct gaze toward the oncoming visual scene
Smooth pursuit	To hold the image of a small moving target on the fovea
Optokinetic	To hold images of the seen world steady on the retina during sustained head rotation
Vestibular	To hold images of the seen world steady (vestibulo-ocular reflex) on the retina during brief head rotations
Vergence	To move the eyes in opposite directions so that images of a single object are placed on both foveas

Modified from Leigh RJ, Zee DS. *The Neurology of Eye Movements*. 3rd ed. New York, NY: Oxford University Press; 1999.

    c. After the eyes have achieved macular fixation of a slowly, smoothly moving target, the eyes will pursue at the velocity of target in a smooth fashion

    d. If the target is moving at a velocity greater than 50°/second, then the eyes, after falling behind in their pursuit, will execute saccadic voluntary FEM in order to regain macular fixation; the eyes will then pursue with the smooth SEM until they fall behind again; this results in another "catch-up" saccadic FEM as in the phenomenon of cogwheel pursuit

    e. Visual fixation—holds the image of a stationary object on the fovea

        i. Special type of smooth pursuit or possibly an independent system

        ii. Detects unwanted drifts of eyes and suppresses saccades

D. SEM: optokinetic system

    1. Stimulus: sustained head rotation

    2. The vestibular system responds only to acceleration. With sustained head rotation at a constant velocity, the vestibular response fades and the optokinetic system supplements visually driven compensatory slow-phase eye movements

E. SEM: vestibular

    1. The membranous labyrinth lies within its bony compartment in the temporal bone, cushioned by perilymph (Figure 2-1)

    2. It contains:

        a. Three semicircular canals and their respective cristae (each in an ampulla), which sense head rotation and measure angular acceleration

        b. The utricle and saccule (otolith organs) and their respective maculae, which sense head position and measure linear acceleration

    3. The semicircular canals, utricle, and saccule contain endolymph

    4. The cristae and maculae contain specialized hair cells that transduce mechanical shearing forces into neural impulses

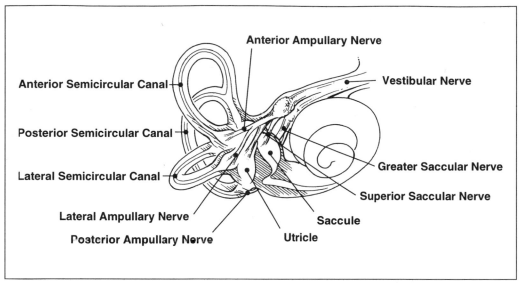

Figure 2-1. Diagram of the membranous inner ear.

  5. The vestibular motion sensors detect transient head rotation
  6. Stimulation of each set of semicircular canals precisely influences a particular pair of eye muscles, thus producing eye movement in a specific direction:
     a. Horizontal canals—horizontal (ipsilateral: medial rectus; contralateral: lateral rectus)
     b. Posterior canals—downward and torsional (ipsilateral: superior oblique; contralateral: inferior rectus)
     c. Anterior canals—upward and torsional (ipsilateral: superior rectus; contralateral: inferior oblique)
  7. The horizontal semicircular canals are oriented 30 degrees above the horizontal, with the ampullae anteriorly located (Figure 2-2)
  8. To maximally affect the horizontal semicircular canals, a specific head position is required (Figure 2-3)
     a. Head is inclined forward 30 degrees for maximal effect of rotational forces in Barany chair (30 degrees above supine position)
     b. Head is inclined backward 60 degrees for maximal effect for the convection currents of endolymph flow with caloric testing (Figures 2-3 and 2-4)
  9. During doll's eye testing, when the head is rotated toward the left side, the endolymph moves toward the left ampulla and away from the right ampulla (Figure 2-5)
 10. Converse movements of the endolymph occur when the head is rotated to the right side
 11. Movement of the endolymph (by warm water calorics, Barany chair rotation, or doll's eye testing) toward the ampulla results in stimulation of that ampulla
 12. Movement of the endolymph (by cold water calorics) away from the ampulla results in inhibition of that ampulla
F. SEM: vergence
    1. Vergence eye movements are disconjugate; they carry the eyes in opposite directions to direct both foveas at one object of interest

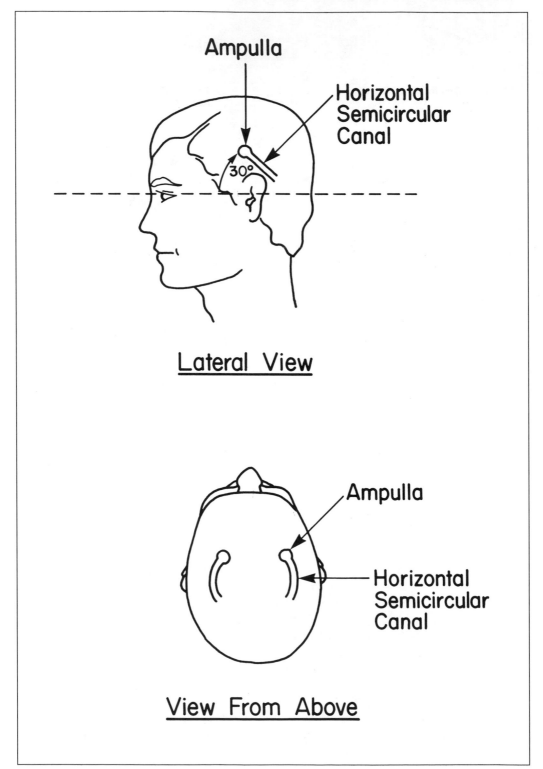

Figure 2-2. Orientation of the horizontal semicircular canals.

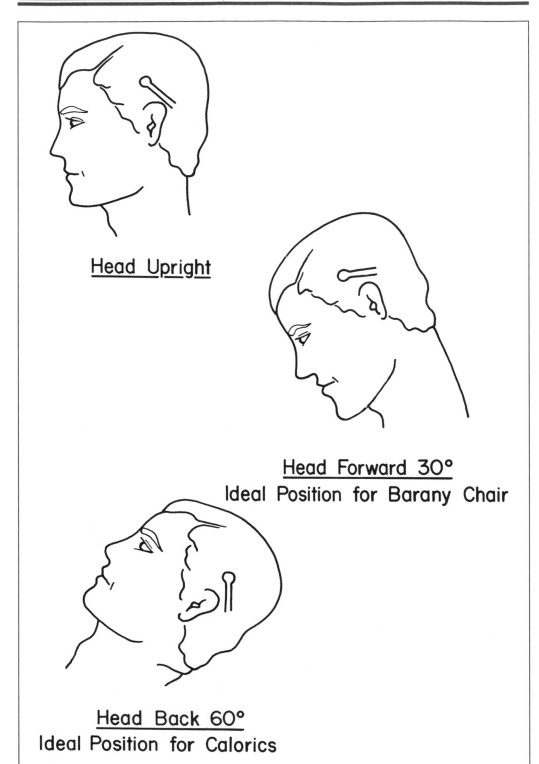

Head Upright

Head Forward 30°
Ideal Position for Barany Chair

Head Back 60°
Ideal Position for Calorics

Figure 2-3.

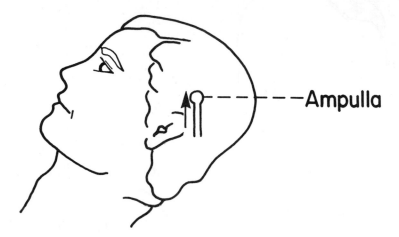

WARM WATER CALORICS: The endolymph rises (arrow) toward the ampulla

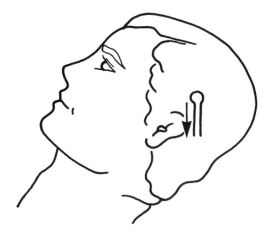

COLD WATER CALORICS: The endolymph falls away from (arrow) the ampulla

Figure 2-4.

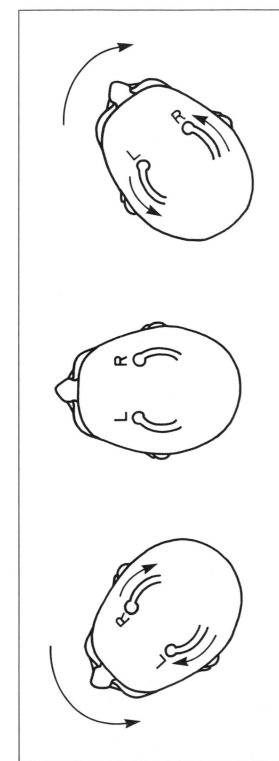

DOLL'S EYE TESTING: When the head is rotated to the left, the endolymph moves toward the left ampulla and away from the right ampulla. When the head is rotated to the right, the endolymph moves toward the right ampulla and away from the left ampulla.

Figure 2-5.

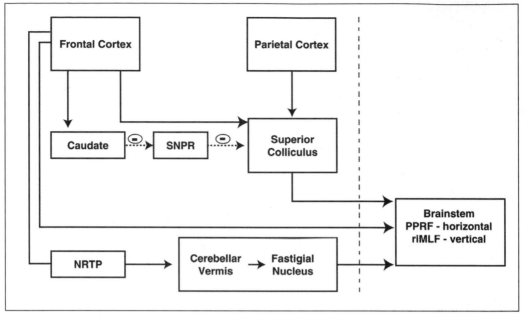

Figure 2-6. Saccadic eye movement pathways. Both direct and multisynaptic pathways lead to generation of saccades. SNPR: substantia nigra, pons reticulata. NRTP: nucleus reticularis tegmenti pontis. Vertical dash line represents midline.

2. Stimuli
    a. Disparity between the location of images on the retina of each eye. This leads to fusional vergence
    b. Loss of focus of images on the retina (retinal blur). This leads to accommodative vergence
3. Vergence movements occur as a synkinesis with accommodation of the lens and pupillary constriction (the near triad)

III. **Neural pathways for eye movements**
  A. FEM: saccades (Figure 2-6)
    1. Mediated by parallel pathways that converge in the brainstem from:
        a. Frontal cortex—frontal eye field (FEF), supplementary eye field, dorsolateral prefrontal cortex
        b. Posterior parietal cortex
        c. Superior colliculus
    2. Horizontal saccades
        a. Cortical pathways originate in the FEF, which encompasses the lateral part of precentral gyrus and parts of middle frontal and superior frontal gyri
        b. FEF lies in the confluent portion of Brodmann areas 6 and 4, but not 8
        c. Projections from FEF course dorsomedially to pass through the anterior limb of the internal capsule. On their way to the brainstem, most fibers reach the ipsilateral superior colliculus (either directly or via the basal ganglia). Projections from the superior colliculus decussate in the lower midbrain and upper pons and terminate in the PPRF (paramedian pontine reticular formation) in the lower pons

    d. Stimulation of the left FEF results in conjugate movement of the eyes to the right side

    e. Stimulation of the right FEF results in conjugate movement of the eyes to the left side

    f. While the pathway from FEF is involved with self-generated saccades from remembered or learned behavior, the parietal pathway is more concerned with reorienting gaze to new targets appearing in space

  3. Vertical saccades

    a. Cortical pathways descend to the rostral interstitial nucleus of the medial longitudinal fasciculus (riMLF) in the midbrain just rostral to the III nerve nucleus at the junction of the midbrain and thalamus

    b. Bilateral stimulation of FEF is required to elicit purely vertical saccades

B. FEM: nystagmus quick phases

  1. Originate in PPRF and riMLF

  2. This phylogenetically old quick-phase system appears to share the same anatomic substrate as the newer voluntary FEM system

C. SEM: smooth pursuit

  1. General agreement is that the parieto-occipito-temporal (P-O-T) junction is an important structure in the cortical control of smooth pursuit

  2. P-O-T junction is confluence of Brodmann areas 19, 37, and 39

  3. Pathways that transmit pursuit commands have a double decussation (Figure 2-7)

  4. Clinically, the system is under ipsilateral control: the right P-O-T junction controls smooth pursuit to the right, and the left junction to the left

  5. A pure occipital lobe lesion, despite the production of a homonymous hemianopia, will not cause deficiency of pursuit eye movements since the pursuit pathways remain intact (Figure 2-8)

  6. Once the half-macula (of the remaining visual field) is able to achieve fixation, the eye is able to pursue the target to either side

  7. General rule: patients with homonymous hemianopia due to optic tract, temporal lobe, or occipital lobe lesions will not have difficulty with smooth pursuit to either side

  8. Deep parietal lobe lesions disrupt optomotor fibers intended for the ipsilateral pons and thereby disrupt smooth pursuit to the ipsilateral side; the patient may still be able to pursue a target to the side ipsilateral of the lesion, but it will be admixed with catch-up saccades, thus exhibiting nonsmooth, cogwheel pursuit (Figure 2-9)

  9. Deep parietal lobe lesions result in asymmetric smooth pursuit, as elicited by the optokinetic drum, when the drum is rotated toward the side of the lesion (see Chapter 1)

  10. Lesion of the P-O-T junction causes akinetopsia, as the patient reports defects of motion perception (see Chapter 18)

D. SEM: optokinetic (OKN) system

  1. Only present when afferent visual pathways to the visual cortex and the connections to the brainstem ocular motor system are intact

  2. Serves as a means of image stabilization to supplement the fading vestibular response of sustained head rotation at a constant velocity

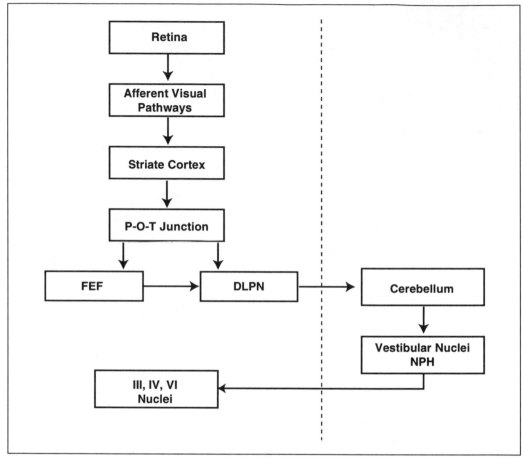

Figure 2-7. Smooth pursuit pathways. Command signal begins in parieto-occipito-temporal (P-O-T) junction, with projections to frontal eye field (FEF) and dorsolateral pontine nuclei (DLPN) in the brainstem. Decussation to the contralateral cerebellum (flocculus, paraflocculus, vermis), then to the vestibular nuclei and nucleus prepositus hypoglossi (NPH); finally, second decussation to the ocular motor (III, IV, I) nuclei. The vertical dash line represents the midline.

3. OKN stabilizes a moving visual field, preventing an otherwise continuous blur from constant relative motion of the visual field
4. Pathways unknown, but the nucleus of the optic tract (in the pretectum) appears important
5. Possibly two neural pathways controlling OKN: subcortical component and phylogenetically newer smooth pursuit component

E. SEM: vestibular (labyrinthine-pontine pathway)
    1. Information from the ampulla of the right horizontal semicircular canal is delivered to the right vestibular nuclear complex. This, in turn, is relayed to the left VI nerve nucleus (horizontal gaze center), resulting in SEM (vestibular) to the left side
    2. Information from the ampulla of the left horizontal semicircular canal arrives at the left vestibular nuclear complex, relayed to the right VI nerve nucleus, resulting in SEM (vestibular) to the right side

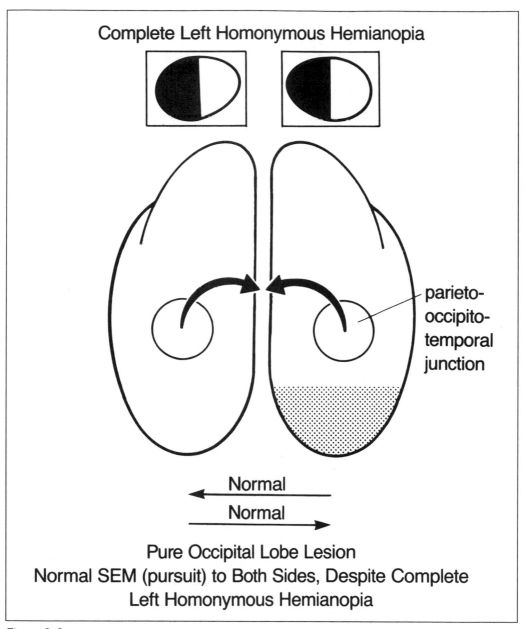

Figure 2-8.

3. Information from the anterior and posterior semicircular canals results in combinations of torsional and vertical eye movements; this probably accounts for the horizontal-torsional nystagmus being a hallmark of labyrinthine disease, involving all three canals on one side

F. SEM: vergence (occipito-mesencephalic pathway)
   1. Disconjugate eye movements enable bifoveal fixation in space from infinity to the near point of convergence

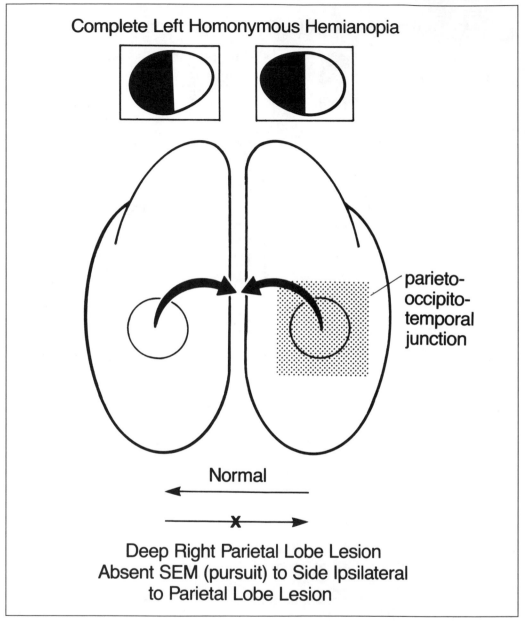

Figure 2-9.

2. The near synkinesis pathway involves occipital cortex and descends to neurons in midbrain reticular formation, dorsal and dorsolateral to the oculomotor nuclei

3. Three types of neurons found in midbrain reticular formation:
   a. Vergence tonic cells—discharge in relation to vergence angle
   b. Vergence burst cells—discharge in relation to vergence velocity
   c. Vergence burst-tonic cells—discharge in relation to both stimuli

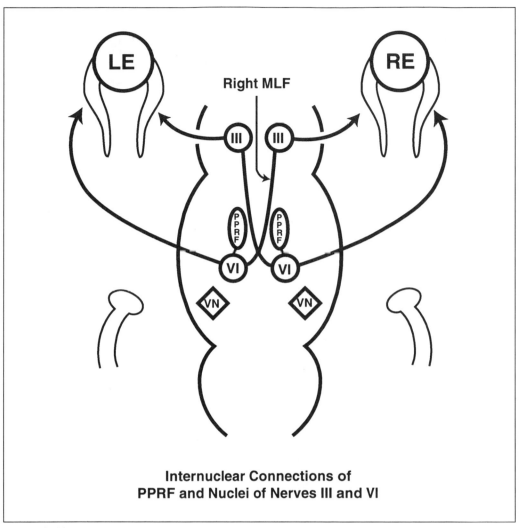

**Internuclear Connections of
PPRF and Nuclei of Nerves III and VI**

Figure 2-10.

> 4. Subsequent specific stimulation of the III nerve nuclear complex leads to the near triad: accommodation, miosis, convergence

IV. Eye movement pathways within the brainstem

A. The neuroanatomy of the brainstem structures involved in eye movements is shown in Figures 2-10 and 2-11

B. As a general rule, horizontal eye movements are generated in the pons and vertical eye movements in the midbrain

C. Horizontal gaze pathways (Figure 2-12)

1. The abducens nucleus is the site of horizontal versional command. The nucleus contains two types of neurons: 1) abducens motoneurons, with axons that innervate the ipsilateral lateral rectus; 2) abducens internuclear neurons, with axons that project through the contralateral medial longitudinal fasciculus to the medial rectus subdivision of the contralateral oculomotor nucleus

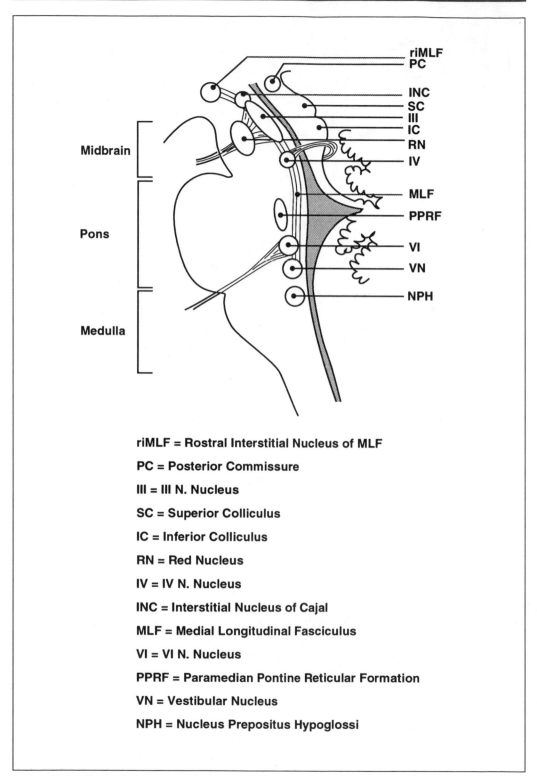

riMLF = Rostral Interstitial Nucleus of MLF

PC = Posterior Commissure

III = III N. Nucleus

SC = Superior Colliculus

IC = Inferior Colliculus

RN = Red Nucleus

IV = IV N. Nucleus

INC = Interstitial Nucleus of Cajal

MLF = Medial Longitudinal Fasciculus

VI = VI N. Nucleus

PPRF = Paramedian Pontine Reticular Formation

VN = Vestibular Nucleus

NPH = Nucleus Prepositus Hypoglossi

Figure 2-11. Sagittal view of the brainstem showing structures important for the generation of horizontal and vertical gaze.

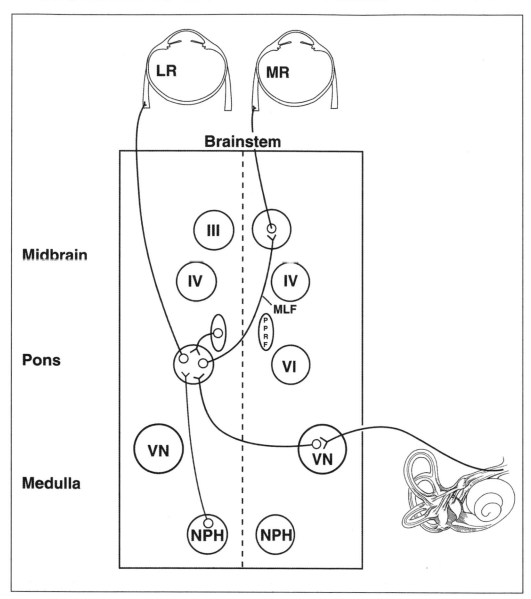

Figure 2-12. Brainstem pathways for horizontal gaze. Axons from cell bodies in the PPRF travel to ipsilateral VI where they synapse with abducens motoneurons, axons of which travel to ipsilateral lateral rectus (LR). Abducens internuclear neurons have axons that cross the midline and travel in the MLF to contact medial rectus (MR) motoneurons in contralateral III. Eye position information (neural integrator) reaches VI from neurons within the nucleus prepositus hypoglossi (NPH) and vestibular nuclei (VN) (modified from Leigh RJ, Zee DS. *The Neurology of Eye Movements.* 3rd ed. New York, NY: Oxford University Press; 1999: 216).

2. Stimulation of the right abducens nucleus causes conjugate gaze to the right, and stimulation of the left abducens nucleus leads to conjugate gaze to the left

3. The PPRF contains cells that project directly to the ipsilateral abducens nucleus

4. The PPRF activates motoneurons during saccadic eye movements

5. The PPRF contains excitatory burst neurons (EBNs) that discharge just prior to a horizontal saccade to stimulate the ipsilateral abducens nucleus. The EBNs are under the inhibitory control of pause neurons that discharge continuously except immediately prior to and during saccades

6. Once the eye has reached a new position, there must be a change in innervation to maintain this eccentric position

7. Tonic gaze-holding mechanism requires a neural network that integrates (in the mathematical sense) velocity-coded signals into position-coded signals. This is referred to as the neural integrator

8. Gaze-holding neural integrator for horizontal gaze includes: 1) medial vestibular nucleus; 2) nucleus prepositus hypoglossi

D. Vertical gaze pathways (Figure 2-13)

1. The rostral interstitial nucleus of the riMLF lies dorsomedial to the red nucleus at the junction of the midbrain and thalamus

2. The riMLF contains excitatory burst neurons for vertical and torsional saccades

3. Efferent information for:

    a. Upward gaze: upward saccadic command from the riMLF projects bilaterally to III nerve nuclei

    b. Downward gaze: downgaze saccadic command projects mainly ipsilaterally to the III and IV cranial nerve nuclei

4. Unilateral activation of the riMLF will generate torsional conjugate eye movements

    a. Stimulate right riMLF—clockwise eye movements (RE: extorts; LE: intorts)

    b. Stimulate left riMLF—counterclockwise eye movements (RE: intorts; LE: extorts)

5. Bilateral activation is necessary for conjugate vertical eye movements

6. Each riMFL receives descending projections from the frontal eye fields, and ascending projections from the vestibular nuclei and PPRF

7. Vertical vestibular and smooth pursuit signals arise from the lower brainstem (pons, medulla)

8. These axons arise from vestibular nucleus neurons and carry signals for eye position and head velocity

9. Axons travel in the MLF

10. Gaze-holding neural integrator for vertical gaze is in the interstitial nucleus of Cajal

V. Vestibularly elicited horizontal eye movements

A. Figure 2-14 shows that the horizontal semicircular canals, at rest, deliver an equal amount of innervation to the contralateral VI nerve nucleus, maintaining a balanced situation for the four horizontal rectus muscles

B. Noncomatose patient

1. When warm water is placed in the right ear, the endolymph moves toward the ampulla of the horizontal canal (see Figure 2-4), causing an increased tone of input received by the left abducens nucleus (Figure 2-15), eventuating in slow conjugate

contraction (vestibular SEM) of the left lateral rectus muscle and the right medial rectus muscle (via the MLF)

2. There will be a compensatory FEM (fast phase) back to the right side, and the combination of left (vestibular) SEM and right (compensatory) FEM produces the clinical phenomenon of right-beating nystagmus following warm water in the right ear

3. Cold water will produce the opposite response, in that the endolymph will now move away from the ampulla of the horizontal canal, causing slow conjugate contraction (vestibular SEM) to the ipsilateral side and a compensatory FEM back to the opposite side (Figure 2-16)

4. J. Lawton Smith, MD has pointed out the usefulness of the mnemonic "COWS" (Cold Opposite; Warm Same) to remind us that, as we have just seen, Warm water in the Right ear results in Right-beating nystagmus; Cold water in the Left ear results in Right-beating nystagmus; Left-beating nystagmus would be produced by Cold water in the Right or Warm water in the Left ear

5. However, note (see Figure 2-15) that the vestibular input produced by the warm water in right ear is responsible not for the FEM (jerk movement of the nystagmus) back to the right, but only for the initial SEM to the left; the mnemonic "COWS" refers to the direction of the jerk component of the calorically induced nystagmus

6. The FEM (jerk component) is actually a compensatory saccadic movement that is seen only in the noncomatose patient who has an intact PPRF

7. Rotational testing for eye movement function in neonates is helpful in determining the state of brainstem pathways for conjugate horizontal gaze

8. Figure 2-17 illustrates the effect of head rotation on right and left horizontal semicircular canals. The infant's eyes tonically deviate in the direction of the movement, with jerk phase of nystagmus toward the opposite side

C. Comatose patient

1. When warm water is placed in the right ear, assuming nuclear and internuclear brainstem connections are intact, there will be slow tonic conjugate movement (vestibular SEM) of the eyes to the left side without compensatory right-jerk nystagmus (the frontopontine connections are nonfunctional in coma). The eyes will remain deviated to the left side for 30 to 60 seconds, then return back to the midline as the symmetrical tone of the semicircular canals is reestablished

2. Similarly, when cold water is placed in the right ear, the patient's eyes will slowly, tonically deviate to the right side, then return to the midline

D. Doll's eye testing with rotation to the head to the right also produces a tonic SEM (vestibular) to the left, provided nuclear and internuclear connections are intact. Figure 2-5 illustrates that this results from a combination of shift of the endolymph away from the left ampulla and toward the right ampulla of the horizontal canals, thereby decreasing the input from the left ampulla and increasing the input from the right ampulla

E. The SEM tone produced by doll's eye testing is not sustained enough to result in compensatory FEM (jerk nystagmus)

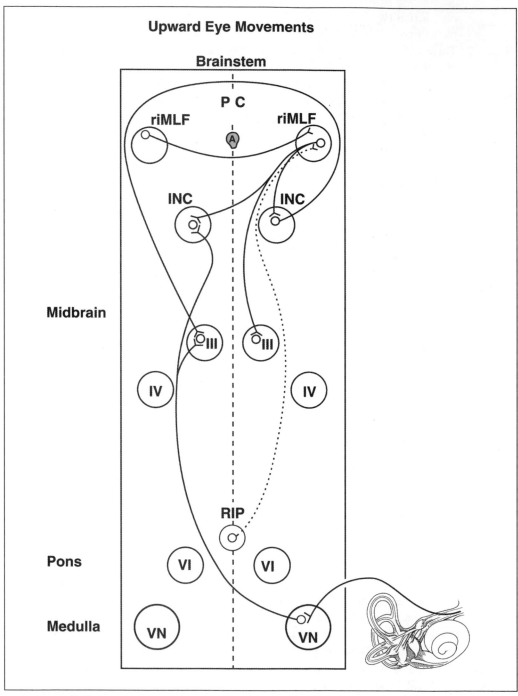

Upward Eye Movements

Figure 2-13 (left). Brainstem pathways for vertical gaze, upward (left) and downward (right, opposite page). Vestibular inputs from the vertical semicircular canals synapse in the vestibular nucleus and ascend in the contralateral MLF and brachium conjunctivum (not shown) to contact neurons in IV, III, interstitial nucleus of Cajal (INC) and riMLF. The riMLF contains saccadic burst neurons and receives an inhibitory input from omnipause neurons of the nucleus raphé interpositus (RIP). Excitatory burst neurons in the riMLF project to III, IV, and send an axon collateral to INC. The INC provides a gaze-holding signal and projects to vertical motoneurons via the posterior commissure (PC). A: aqueduct of Sylvius (modified from Leigh RJ, Zee DS. *The Neurology of Eye Movements.* 3rd ed. New York, NY: Oxford University Press: 1999; 225).

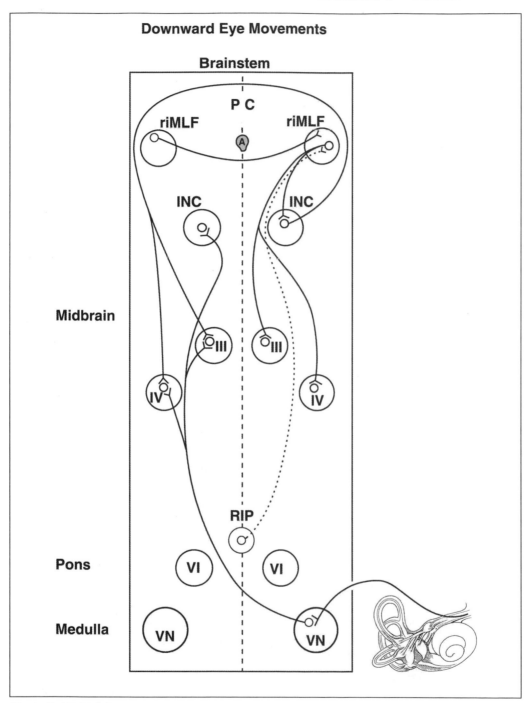

Figure 2-13 (right).

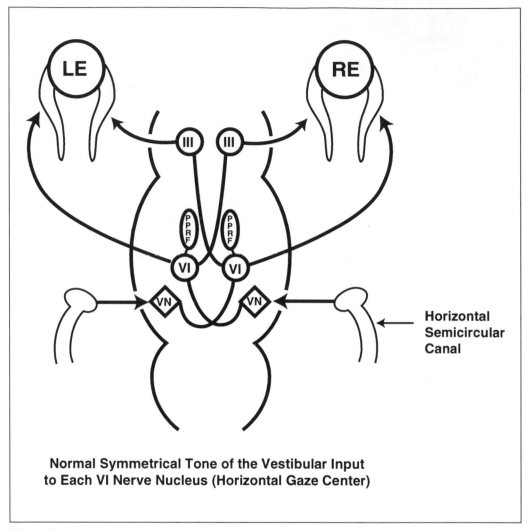

**Normal Symmetrical Tone of the Vestibular Input
to Each VI Nerve Nucleus (Horizontal Gaze Center)**

Figure 2-14.

VI.   Horizontal gaze abnormalities

A. Supranuclear

1. Acute cerebrovascular accident (CVA) affecting frontal or parietal lobes

a. Eyes (and sometimes head) tonically deviate toward the side of the lesion, since the contralateral FEF has unopposed action

b. Doll's eye testing and calorics can turn the eyes contralateral to the lesion (since the SEM [vestibular] pathway is intact), but the eyes then return to tonic deviation toward the lesion

c. Within 3 to 7 days, the patients begin to exhibit voluntary eye movements away from the lesion

2. Congenital ocular motor apraxia

a. Deficiency of voluntary horizontal eye movements

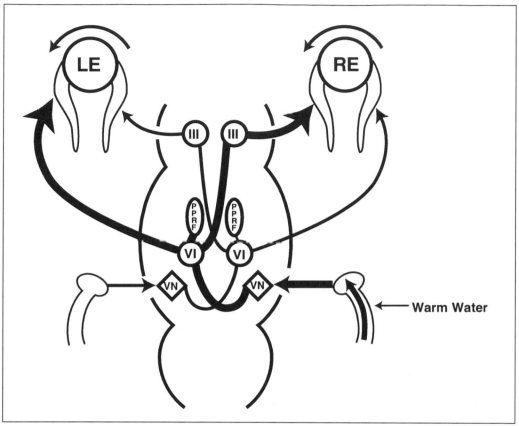

Figure 2-15. Warm water in the right ear causes shift of endolymph toward the ampulla, thereby increasing the vestibular tone and resulting in a slow movement of the eyes to the left side. The compensatory fast phase will be directed back to the right side (COWS).

b. Vertical movements normal; horizontal SEM (vestibular) normal

c. Random saccades and pursuit horizontal eye movements may be seen

d. When the patient seeks to change visual fixation horizontally, he or she does so by "thrusting" the head toward the desired direction of gaze

e. The head movement elicits a contralateral SEM (vestibular), driving the eyes to an extreme contraversive orbital position

f. The head then continues to move past the target (an overshoot), dragging the eyes mechanically in the same direction until they reach the target

g. The patient then straightens his or her head while maintaining fixation on the new target

h. The head movement and "overshoot" produce the phenomenon of head thrusting, which is the hallmark of congenital ocular motor apraxia

i. The head-thrusting becomes less prominent with age

j. Congenital ocular motor apraxia may be associated with CNS disorders such as agenesis of the corpus callosum, collicular abnormalities, cerebellar vermian dysplasia (eg, Joubert syndrome)

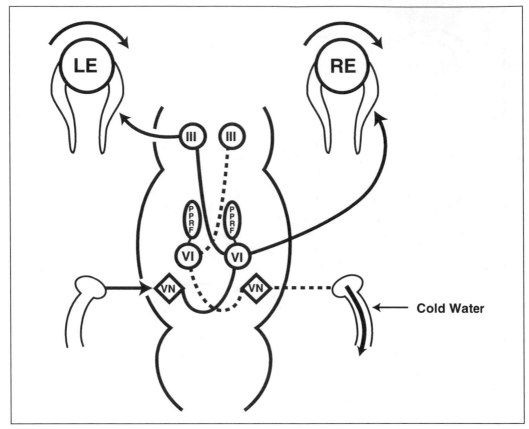

Figure 2-16. Cold water in the right ear causes shift of endolymph away from the ampulla, thereby decreasing the vestibular tone and allowing the vestibular tone from the left side to be dominant. This results in a slow movement of the eyes to the right. The compensatory fast phase will therefore be directed to the left side (COWS).

3. Balint's syndrome: acquired ocular motor apraxia
    a. Patients with extensive bilateral cerebral disease (parieto-occipital) (see Chapter 18)
    b. Difficulty initiating reflexive (visually guided) saccades and SEM (pursuit) in all directions, with intact SEM (vestibular) and relative preservation of volitional saccades
    c. Simultanagnosia—inability to perceive more than one object at a time
    d. Optic ataxia—inaccurate arm pointing
    e. Ocular motor apraxia—difficulty initiating voluntary saccades
    f. Frequently have associated dementia and visual field defects
4. Spasticity of conjugate gaze (Cogan's sign)
    a. A "screening" test for cerebral disease
    b. Normally, during forced lid closure, each eye is deviated superolaterally (Bell's phenomenon)
    c. Patients with lesions of the temporal or parietal lobe may show conjugate deviation of the eye superiorly and away from the side of the lesion

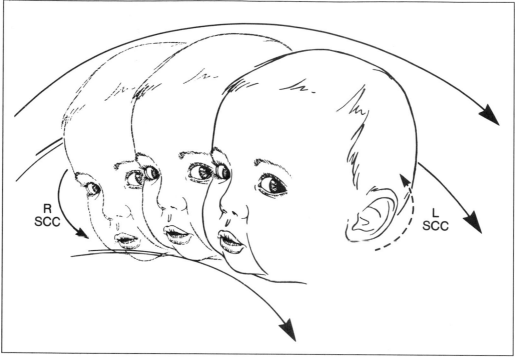

Figure 2-17. Rotational testing for eye movement function in infants. As the infant is spun toward his or her left (toward the examiner's right), the eye will tonically deviate in the direction of the movement with jerk phase of nystagmus toward the opposite side. This leads to stimulation of the right semicircular canals (SCC) and inhibition of the left SCC.

      d. This spasticity of conjugate gaze is not seen with frontal lobe lesions, and the reasons for this are poorly understood

      e. Cogan's sign is of lateralizing but not localizing value

B. Pontine conjugate gaze palsy

    1. Unilateral VI nerve nucleus or PPRF lesion creates an ipsilateral conjugate horizontal gaze palsy

    2. With acute lesions, the eyes may be deviated contralaterally

    3. Ipsilaterally directed saccades and quick phases of nystagmus are small and slow and do not carry the eyes past the midline

    4. With VI nerve nuclear lesions all types of ipsilaterally directed eye movements are abolished

    5. Smooth pursuit and slow phases of OKN may be preserved in both directions within the intact field of movement but cannot bring the eyes past the midline

    6. In patients with isolated PPRF lesions, vestibular stimuli (eg, calorics) drive the eyes across the midline. Presumably, the ipsilateral abducens nucleus and its direct vestibular input are intact, and the PPRF lesion causing the horizontal gaze palsy is more rostral

C. Internuclear ophthalmoplegia (INO)

    1. A lesion of the MLF blocks information from the contralateral VI nerve nucleus to the ipsilateral III nerve nucleus (Figure 2-18); this "internuclear" lesion results in the clinical phenomenon of an INO

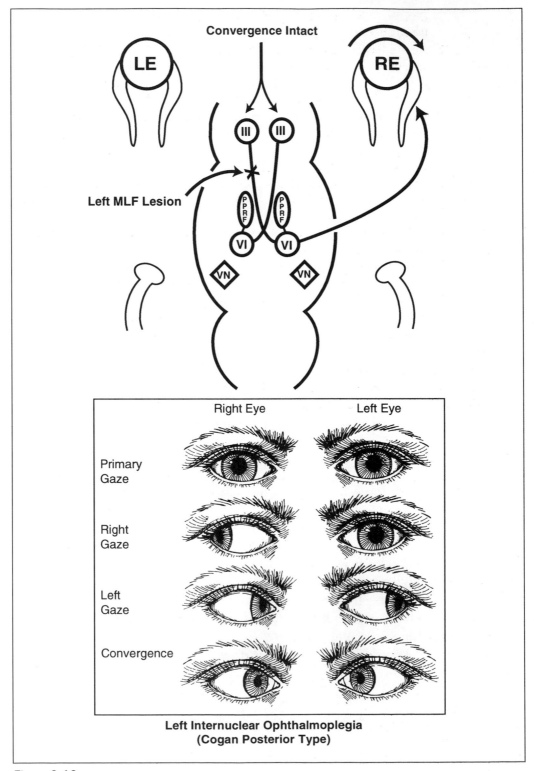

Left Internuclear Ophthalmoplegia
(Cogan Posterior Type)

Figure 2-18.

    a. Deficient adduction during attempted conjugate gaze away from the side of the MLF lesion

    b. Abduction nystagmus (ie, nystagmus of the abducting eye during attempted conjugate gaze away from the side of the lesion)

    c. An MLF lesion is on the same side as the eye with the medial rectus (adduction) weakness. INO is named for the side of the MLF lesion

    d. Usually medial rectus function is better preserved when convergence is stimulated (Cogan's posterior INO)

    e. INO produced by a mesencephalic lesion is usually bilateral and may have an absence of convergence (Cogan's anterior INO)

    f. Unilateral or bilateral INO in a young adult is most likely due to multiple sclerosis; whereas a unilateral INO in a patient over age 50 is most likely due to brainstem vascular disease

    g. WEBINO (wall-eyed bilateral INO) syndrome refers to an exotropic patient who has bilateral INOs. It is impossible to exclude involvement of the medial rectus subnuclei, as well as both MLFs, unless convergence is preserved

    h. INO may be accompanied by skew deviation with the eye ipsilateral to the lesion being hypertropic. There may also be disconjugate vertical nystagmus

    i. Bilateral INOs are often seen with vertical gaze-evoked nystagmus, due to impairment of vertical pursuit and vestibular signals (see Section IV, D)

  D. One-and-a-half syndrome

    1. Lesion of the VI nerve nucleus or PPRF and ipsilateral MLF (Figure 2-19)

    2. Pontine conjugate gaze palsy to the ipsilateral side ("one")

    3. INO on gaze to the contralateral side (the "half")

  E. Paralytic pontine exotropia

    1. A transient phenomenon seen in one-and-a-half syndrome during the first few days after onset

    2. The VI nerve nucleus or PPRF lesion causes the contralateral VI nerve nucleus or PPRF to be unopposed; therefore, the eyes tend to deviate conjugately away from the lesion

    3. However, because of the INO, the ipsilateral eye cannot adduct

    4. The eye contralateral to the MLF lesion remains tonically abducted and demonstrates an exotropia

VII. Vertical gaze abnormalities

  A. Downgaze palsy—due to midbrain disease (stroke, tumor) with lesions involving the riMLF just rostral to the III nerve nucleus and dorsomedially to the red nucleus

  B. Upgaze palsy—association with lesions located more dorsally, contiguous with the posterior commissure

  C. Dorsal midbrain syndrome

    1. Also known as "pretectal syndrome," "Sylvian aqueduct syndrome," or "Parinaud's syndrome"

    2. Supranuclear paresis of vertical gaze: vertical FEM and vertical SEM (smooth pursuit and vestibular) are variably affected, mainly in upward direction, reflecting involvement of INC and its projections

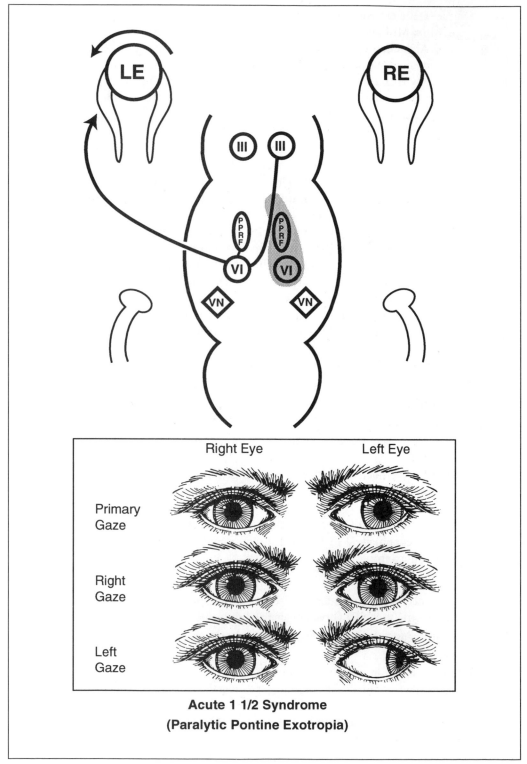

Acute 1 1/2 Syndrome
(Paralytic Pontine Exotropia)

Figure 2-19.

3. Other associated eye signs
    a. Light-near dissociation of the pupils
    b. Convergence-retraction nystagmus
    c. Lid retraction (Collier's sign)
    d. Spasm/paresis of convergence
    e. Spasm/paresis of accommodation
    f. Skew deviation (see Section IX)

D. Monocular elevation paresis
    1. No abnormality in primary position or looking down, but diplopia in upgaze due to limitation of elevation in one eye
    2. Associated pupillary abnormality that may include anisocoria, sluggish light reaction, and light-near dissociation
    3. Forced ductions and Tensilon testing are both negative
    4. Presumed interruption of supranuclear input from riMLF (mediating upgaze) to III nerve nucleus

E. Progressive supranuclear palsy
    1. Steele-Richardson-Olszewski syndrome
    2. Progressive conjugate paresis of gaze in all directions, but usually affecting vertical saccades (especially downward) initially
    3. SEM are initially preserved, vestibular more than pursuit
    4. Some clinical features similar to Parkinsonism
        a. Nuchal dystonic rigidity
        b. Seborrheic skin changes
        c. Usually no resting tremor
    5. Characterized by recurrent falls early in the course
    6. Progressive dementia and death usually within 5 years

F. Oculogyric crisis
    1. Tonic vertical or horizontal supranuclear deviation of the eyes; able to overcome with SEM (vestibular), but eyes then return to the tonically deviated position
    2. Seen with postencephalitic Parkinsonism and neuroleptic toxicity

VIII. Disorders of vergence

A. Spasm of the near reflex
    1. Triad of convergence, accommodation, miosis
    2. May simulate unilateral or bilateral VI nerve palsies
    3. Usually psychogenic, as patient presents with variable esotropia
    4. Rarely due to organic disease: head trauma, dorsal midbrain syndrome, intoxication, Wernicke's encephalopathy

B. Convergence paresis/paralysis
    1. Patients report diplopia at near or easy fatigability while reading
    2. Usual causes: aging, lack of effort
    3. Rarely due to organic cause: dorsal midbrain syndrome, multiple sclerosis, encephalitis, diphtheria, botulism

C. Divergence paresis/paralysis

1. Clinical syndrome characterized by:
   a. Orthophoria at near
   b. Comitant esotropia at distance
   c. Full extraocular movements
2. May present in adult with no other neurologic findings/dysfunction
3. Must exclude:
   a. Decompensated esophoria
   b. Subtle bilateral VI nerve palsies
4. May be seen in a variety of settings: head trauma, progressive supranuclear palsy, brainstem stroke, seizure disorder, Arnold-Chiari I malformation

IX.   Skew deviation

A. An acquired vertical and torsional ocular deviation from supranuclear dysfunction

B. Due to imbalance of otolithic inputs to ocular motor neurons from utricle and saccule up to INC. Represents part of ocular tilt reaction (see below)

C. May be comitant or noncomitant

D. May be seen with internuclear ophthalmoplegia and/or vertical gaze-evoked nystagmus

E. Caused by a lesion anywhere in the midbrain, pons, medulla, vestibular nerve or inner ear: infarction, tumor, trauma, multiple sclerosis

F. With lower brainstem lesions, the eye ipsilateral to the lesion tends to be hypotropic; with pontine and midbrain lesions, the ipsilateral eye tends to be hypertropic

X.   Ocular tilt reaction (OTR)

A. OTR is a disorder of head and gaze stabilization

B. Due to lesion affecting peripheral (utricular) or central otolithic pathways (vestibular nuclei, MLF, INC)

C. Stimulation of INC leads to:
   1. Ipsilateral head tilt
   2. Depression and extorsion of ipsilateral eye
   3. Elevation and intorsion of contralateral eye

D. Destructive lesion of INC leads to:
   1. Contralateral head tilt
   2. Elevation and intorsion of ipsilateral eye
   3. Depression and extorsion of contralateral eye

E. Clinically, a destructive lesion (tumor, trauma, demyelination, infarction) causing OTR can mimic a three-step test of IV nerve palsy. Differentiation with measurement of torsion:
   1. IV nerve palsy—extorsion of hypertropic eye
   2. OTR—intorsion of hypertropic eye

F. Usually resolves within months, with restoration of normal head and eye position

XI.   Ocular neuromyotonia

A. Patient reports episodic diplopia or oscillopsia

B. Failure of extraocular muscles to "relax" following sustained, eccentric gaze

C. Previous history of invasive pituitary adenoma or other intracranial tumors treated with radiation therapy

D. Due to episodic, involuntary discharge of ocular motor nerves producing sustained and inappropriate contraction of their respective ocular muscles

E. Treatment: carbamazepine, phenytoin

XII. Wernicke's encephalopathy

A. Triad: ophthalmoplegia, mental confusion, gait ataxia

B. Ocular motor findings include: abduction weakness, gaze-evoked nystagmus, internuclear ophthalmoplegia, upbeat nystagmus, impaired vestibulo-ocular reflex, horizontal and vertical gaze palsies that may progress to total ophthalmoplegia

C. Ophthalmoplegia bilateral but may be asymmetric

D. Lesions occur throughout brainstem, thalamus, hypothalamus, and cerebellum

E. Due to thiamine B_1 deficiency

F. Most commonly seen in alcoholics

G. Treatment with thiamine

H. Korsakoff's syndrome is more severe thiamine-deficiency encephalopathy with memory loss and permanent ocular motor abnormalities

BIBLIOGRAPHY

Books

Büttner U, Brandt T. Ocular motor disorders of the brainstem. In: Büttner U, Brandt T. *Balliere's Clinical Neurology.* Philadelphia, Pa: Balliere Tindoll; 1992.

Leigh RJ, Zee DS. *The Neurology of Eye Movements.* 3rd ed. New York, NY: Oxford University Press; 1999.

Chapters

Leigh RJ, Daroff RB, Troost BT. Supranuclear disorders of eye movements. In: Glaser JS, ed. *Neuro-ophthalmology.* 3rd ed. Philadelphia, Pa: Lippincott-Williams & Wilkins; 1999: 345-368.

Sharpe JA. Neural control of ocular motor systems. In: Miller NR, Newman NJ, eds. *Walsh and Hoyt's Clinical Neuro-ophthalmology.* Vol 1. 5th ed. Baltimore, Md: Williams & Wilkins; 1998: 1101-1167.

Zee DS. Supranuclear and internuclear ocular motor disorders. In: Miller NR, Newman NJ, eds. *Walsh and Hoyt's Clinical Neuro-ophthalmology.* 5th ed. Vol 1. Baltimore, Md: Williams & Wilkins; 1998: 1283-1349.

Articles

Baker RS, Epstein AD. Ocular motor abnormalities from head trauma. *Surv Ophthalmol.* 1991;35:245-267.

Cogan DG. Congenital ocular motor apraxia. *Can J Ophthalmol.* 1966;1:253-260.

Cogan DG. Paralysis of down-gaze. *Arch Ophthalmol.* 1974;91:192-199.

Donahue SP, Lavin PJ, Hamed LM. Tonic ocular tilt reaction simulating a superior oblique palsy. Diagnostic confusion with the three-step test. *Arch Ophthalmol.* 1999;117:347-352.

Fisher CM. Some neuro-ophthalmological observations. *J Neurol Neurosurg Psychiatry.* 1967;30:383-392.

Green JP, Newman NJ, Winterkorn JS. Paralysis of downgaze in two patients with clinical-radiologic correlation. *Arch Ophthalmol.* 1993;111:219-222.

Keane JR. Ocular skew deviation. *Arch Neurol.* 1975;32:185-190.

Leigh RJ, Brandt T. A re-evaluation of the vestibular-ocular reflex. *Neurology.* 1993;43:1288-1295.

Pola J, Robinson DA. An explanation of eye movements seen in internuclear ophthalmoplegia. *Arch Neurol.* 1976;33:447-452.

Shults WT, Hoyt WF, Behrens MM, et al. Ocular neuromytonia. *Arch Ophthalmol.* 1986;104:1028-1034.

Smith JL, Gay AJ, Cogan DG. The spasticity of conjugate gaze phenomenon. *Arch Ophthalmol.* 1959; 62:694-696.

Steele JC, Richardson JC, Olszewski J. Progressive supranuclear palsy: a heterogeneous degeneration involving the brain stem, basal ganglia and cerebellum with vertical gaze and pseudobulbar palsy, nuchal dystonia and dementia. *Arch Neurol.* 1964;1:333-359.

Trojanowski JQ, Wray SH. Vertical gaze ophthalmoplegia: selective paralysis of downgaze. *Neurology.* 1980;30:605-610.

Chapter 3

Nystagmus and Related Ocular Oscillations

I. **Definition: rhythmic, involuntary to-and-fro oscillation of the eyes**

II. **Nystagmus jargon**

   A. Type
   1. Pendular: phases of equal velocity
   2. Jerk: phases of unequal velocity

   B. Direction: the direction of the fast component. The pathological movement, however, is the slow one

   C. Trajectory: horizontal, vertical, diagonal, rotary, circular, elliptical

   D. Amplitude: fine, medium, coarse

   E. Frequency: rapid, slow

   F. Dissociated: nystagmus is of different amplitude between the two eyes

   G. Conjugacy: conjugate if both eyes demonstrate same movement; disconjugate if the eyes have different movements (eg, one eye has horizontal nystagmus and the other circular, or the eyes are not in phase)

   H. Alexander's law: jerk nystagmus usually increases in amplitude with gaze in the direction of the fast phase

   I. Null zone: that field of gaze in which the nystagmus intensity is minimal

   J. Neutral zone: that field of gaze in which bilateral jerk nystagmus reverses direction

   K. Nystagmus is due to an abnormality of the SEM system. Three types of wave forms using eye movement recordings include: increasing velocity exponential slow phase, decreasing velocity exponential slow phase, and linear velocity slow phase

III. **Congenital nystagmus and afferent visual system disorders**

   A. Traditional description of two forms of congenital nystagmus is no longer valid
   1. Afferent nystagmus—nystagmus due to poor vision
   2. Efferent nystagmus—nystagmus due to ocular motor disturbance

   B. Causes of poor vision early in life include:

1. Ocular albinism
2. Aniridia
3. Achromatopsia
4. Congenital optic nerve disease: atrophy, hypoplasia
5. Congenital cataracts

C. On the basis of eye movement recordings, congenital nystagmus associated with poor visual function cannot be distinguished from congenital nystagmus without afferent visual system dysfunction

D. Therefore, congenital nystagmus is conceptualized as primary motor disturbance

E. Nystagmus secondary to visual loss can only be diagnosed if it is known that the nystagmus developed after the visual problem began; otherwise, the nystagmus may coexist with the visual disturbance, but a causal relationship cannot be assumed

IV. Clinical classification of nystagmus

A. Physiologic nystagmus

B. Specific, recognizable, localizing types of nystagmus

C. Gaze-evoked nystagmus

D. Related oscillations

V. Physiologic nystagmus

A. End-position nystagmus—three forms
1. Fatigue nystagmus: occurs after prolonged (10 to 15 seconds) deviation of eyes
2. Unsustained end-position nystagmus: seen initially at extremes of gaze (except downgaze) but resolves in 5 to 10 seconds
3. Sustained end-position nystagmus: symmetric, fine nystagmus in extreme right and left gaze; disappears when gaze returns back toward primary position

B. Optokinetic nystagmus (OKN)
1. OKN allows image stabilization when viewing a consistently moving visual field (see Chapter 2)
2. OKN can be conceptualized simplistically as a combination of SEM (pursuit) and compensatory FEM (saccade) to pick up fixation of the next target on the OKN stimulus
3. OKN is abnormal when it is "asymmetric": greater OKN demonstrated when target is moving in one direction compared to the opposite
4. Asymmetric OKN (diminished OKN when target is moving toward side of the lesion) may be seen in association with homonymous hemianopia due to a deep parietal lesion (see Chapters 1 and 2)
5. However, a homonymous hemianopia alone does not cause the diminished OKN; normal OKN is seen in a patient with hemianopia due to optic tract, temporal lobe, and occipital lobe lesions
6. OKN test of vision: can substantiate the presence of vision in a patient with functional blindness (see Chapter 17)

C. Caloric nystagmus (see Chapter 2)
1. Combination of SEM (vestibular) and compensatory FEM (saccade)
2. Vestibular SEM elicited by stimulation (shift of endolymph toward ampulla) or inhibition (shift of endolymph away from ampulla) of one or more semicircular canals

    3. Unilateral irrigation produces nystagmus, which is either horizontal, rotary, or oblique depending on the position of the head

    4. Bilateral simultaneous caloric stimulation produces vertical nystagmus: CUWD (cold, up; warm, down—direction of fast phase of nystagmus)

D. Rotational nystagmus (see Figure 2-5)

    1. Rotating or accelerating head movements induce movement of endolymph in the semicircular canals, which results in jerk nystagmus

    2. During rotation, the eyes tonically deviate in the direction of the movement

    3. Nystagmus quick phases are toward the opposite side

    4. Useful in the evaluation of the ocular motor system in infants (see Figure 2-17)

VI. Specific, recognizable, localizing types of nystagmus

A. Congenital nystagmus

    1. May be present at birth or appear later within the perinatal period

    2. May be sporadic or follow X-linked, autosomal dominant, or autosomal recessive inheritance pattern

    3. Chromosome 6p12 is the first reported genetic locus for autosomal dominant congenital nystagmus

    4. Congenital nystagmus is usually of horizontal form but may be vertical, circular, or elliptical; it may be pendular or jerk

    5. Characterized by pendular or increasing velocity exponential slow phase on eye movement recordings

    6. Dell'Osso and Daroff list 11 characteristics of congenital nystagmus:

        a. Binocular and conjugate

        b. Similar amplitude in both eyes (associated)

        c. No oscillopsia (illusion of environmental movement)

        d. Abolished in sleep

        e. May have associated head oscillation

        f. Damped by convergence

        g. Increased by fixation effort and anxiety

        h. May have superimposed latent nystagmus (see B, Latent nystagmus, next page)

        i. Inversion of the optokinetic reflex: induced nystagmus in the opposite direction to that expected

        j. Distinctive wave forms with eye movement recording: increasing velocity exponential of the slow phase or pendular

        k. Uniplanar: hallmark of congenital nystagmus. Plane of the nystagmus, usually horizontal, remains unchanged in all positions of gaze, including vertical gaze. This phenomenon is seen in only three entities:

            i. Congenital nystagmus

            ii. Peripheral vestibular nystagmus

            iii. Periodic alternating nystagmus

        7. Can frequently identify a null zone of gaze in which the nystagmus is least marked and the visual acuity is best

        8. Patient may manifest head turn to keep the eyes in a null zone; may require muscle surgery (Kestenbaum procedure) in order to place the null zone in the primary position

9. High astigmatism frequently found

10. Nystagmus is usually damped by convergence, so the patient usually has good near acuity and can do well in school

11. Patients may be helped by contact lenses to correct the astigmatism and obviate the visual aberrations created by an eye wiggling behind a spectacle lens that has a high astigmatic correction

12. Patients may also be helped by base-out prism glasses that induce convergence (with its nystagmus damping effect) during distance fixation

B. Latent nystagmus

1. Nystagmus seen only when one eye is covered

2. The patient develops bilateral jerk nystagmus with the jerk component directed away from the covered eye

3. Has linear or decreasing velocity exponential slow phase on eye movement recordings

4. Visual acuity diminished (due to nystagmus) when each eye is tested separately; acuity improves when both eyes are uncovered

5. May coexist with ongoing primary position pendular, jerk, or torsional nystagmus, which converts to latent nystagmus pattern following monocular occlusion

6. This type of nystagmus is congenital and may be seen in association with dissociated vertical deviation and strabismus (usually esotropia)

C. Manifest latent nystagmus

1. Present with both eyes open but only one used for vision (other one suppressed; eg, strabismus or amblyopia)

2. Low intensity jerk nystagmus with the fast phase in the direction of the viewing eye

3. Patients may have their face turned toward the direction of the fast component (eyes turn in opposite direction) with improvement of vision

4. Slow phase is decreasing velocity exponential

D. Spasmus nutans

1. Triad of head turn, head nodding, and nystagmus

2. Begins in first 18 months of life and resolves within first decade of life

3. Horizontal or vertical, pendular, low amplitude, high frequency nystagmus

4. May be unilateral or of different amplitude in each eye; amplitude and phase relationship between eyes is highly variable

5. Acquired monocular nystagmus has been reported as initial sign of anterior visual pathway glioma

6. Therefore, spasmus nutans is a diagnosis of exclusion requiring magnetic resonance (MR) scanning to exclude anterior visual pathway pathology

E. Dissociated and disconjugate nystagmus

1. The nystagmus in one eye is different than the other

2. Different direction: for example, one eye has vertical and the other eye has horizontal nystagmus (disconjugate)

3. See-saw nystagmus (see below) is an example of disconjugate nystagmus

4. Different amplitude: one eye demonstrates greater amplitude than the other (dissociated)

5. The abduction nystagmus of internuclear ophthalmoplegia (INO) is an example of dissociated nystagmus

F. Downbeat nystagmus
   1. Fast phase down while the eyes are in primary position of gaze
   2. Downbeat nystagmus often accentuated during lateral downgaze
   3. Usually associated with lesion at the craniocervical junction (at the level of the foramen magnum)
       a. Arnold-Chiari malformation
       b. Platybasia
       c. Paget's disease
   4. Variety of other causes:
       a. Cerebellar degeneration
       b. Brainstem stroke
       c. Multiple sclerosis
       d. Cerebellar tumor
       e. Head trauma
       f. Increased intracerebral pressure with hydrocephalus
       g. Toxic-metabolic
           i.   Lithium
           ii. Anticonvulsants
           iii. Magnesium deficiency
           iv. Vitamin B_{12} deficiency
           v.   Wernicke's encephalopathy
       h. Congenital
G. Upbeat nystagmus
   1. Fast phase up while the eyes are in primary position of gaze; upbeating during lateral gaze as well
   2. May be of large or small amplitude
   3. Reported causes include:
       a. Cerebellar degeneration
       b. Multiple sclerosis
       c. Brainstem stroke
       d. Posterior fossa tumor
       e. Brainstem encephalitis
       f. Wernicke's encephalopathy
       g. Congenital
H. See-saw nystagmus
   1. Pendular
   2. Conjugate—torsional with disconjugate vertical component
   3. One eye elevates and intorts; the other depresses and extorts
   4. Frequently associated with suprasellar mass lesion, bitemporal hemianopia, visual loss
   5. Other reported etiologies:
       a. Midbrain stroke
       b. Multiple sclerosis
       c. Arnold-Chiari malformation
       d. Head trauma

e. Congenital

    i. Rarely reversed pattern (elevation and extorsion, depression and intorsion)

    ii. Reported with retnitis pigmentosa, albinism, optic nerve hypoplasia

I. Convergence-retraction nystagmus

  1. Jerk convergence-retraction movements due to cocontraction of the extraocular muscles, especially on attempted convergence or upward gaze

  2. Dorsal midbrain syndrome (Sylvian aqueduct, pretectal, Parinaud's syndrome)

    a. Defective vertical gaze, especially upward

    b. Light-near dissociation of the pupils

    c. Lid retraction (Collier's sign)

    d. Convergence-retraction nystagmus

    e. Spasm/paresis of convergence

    f. Spasm/paresis of accommodation

    g. Skew deviation

  3. The convergence-retraction nystagmus is best seen during testing of the eyes with down-going OKN targets, which require upward saccades

  4. J. Lawton Smith, MD suggested an age differential of possible etiologies:

    a. 0 (infant): congenital aqueductal stenosis

    b. 10-year-old: pinealoma

    c. 20-year-old: head trauma

    d. 30-year-old: brainstem vascular malformation

    e. 40-year-old: multiple sclerosis

    f. 50-year-old: basilar artery stroke

J. Periodic alternating nystagmus (PAN)

  1. Jerk nystagmus while eyes are in primary position with the fast component to one side for about 2 minutes, followed by fast component to the other side lasting about 2 minutes

  2. This cycle repeats continuously every 4 minutes

  3. Nystagmus remains horizontal in vertical gaze (uniplanar)

  4. May be accompanied by periodic head rotations to partially or completely null the nystagmus

  5. Etiologies

    a. Congenital

    b. Vesibulocerebellar disease: stroke, multiple sclerosis, spinocerebellar degeneration, Arnold-Chiari malformation

    c. Severe, acquired bilateral visual loss (optic atrophy, vitreous hemorrhage)

    d. Anticonvulsant therapy

    e. Creutzfeldt-Jakob disease

  6. Correction of visual loss (vitrectomy, cataract surgery) may abolish nystagmus

K. Vestibular nystagmus

  1. Due to dysfunction of the vestibular end-organ, nerve nuclear complex, or brainstem connections

  2. Peripheral vestibular nystagmus

a. Nystagmus characteristics
   i. Mixed directional; usually a horizontal-torsional, primary position jerk nystagmus
   ii. Nystagmus of greatest amplitude when gaze is in the direction of the fast component (Alexander's law)
   iii. Almost invariably has a torsional component
   iv. Uniplanar, with linear velocity slow phase on oculography
   v. Suppressed by visual fixation; increased when fixation removed
b. Fast phase usually beats away from the damaged end-organ
c. Frequently associated with vertigo, tinnitus, deafness
d. Labyrinthine disease usually causes suppression of labyrinthine input, thereby simulating the symptoms caused by cold water calorics; thus, cold water in the left ear of a normal subject reproduces the symptoms of left labyrinthine disease
   i. Nystagmus fast-phase to right (COWS)
   ii. The slow component is to the left; therefore, the environment appears to move to the right
   iii. The subject past-points to the left
   iv. Romberg falls to the left when head is in primary position; Romberg falls backward when the face is turned to the left; Romberg falls forward when the face is turned to the right
e. Etiologies
   i. Labyrinthitis
   ii. Neuritis
   iii. Meniere's disease
   iv. Vascular ischemia
   v. Traumatic
   vi. Toxic
   vii. Benign paroxysmal positional vertigo
f. Resolves within days or weeks due to:
   i. Central compensation of asymmetric vestibular input
   ii. Visual suppression
g. Tullio phenomenon: rarely noises induce peripheral vestibular nystagmus
3. Central vestibular nystagmus: see downbeat (Section VI, F), upbeat (Section VI, G) and PAN (Section VI, J)
a. Nystagmus characteristics
   i. Unidirectional
   ii. May be purely vertical or, less frequently, purely horizontal or rotary
   iii. Jerk nystagmus may change direction with change in direction of gaze or upon convergence
   iv. Not greatly influenced by removal of fixation (eg, frenzel high-plus goggles)
   v. Linear, increasing, or decreasing velocity slow phase on oculography
b. Vertigo, tinnitus, deafness are usually less prominent symptoms
c. Romberg direction of fall does not vary with change in head position

   d. Etiology: brainstem dysfunction due to:
      i.   Tumor
      ii. Trauma
      iii. Stroke
      iv. Demyelination
   e. Usually chronic in duration

L. Voluntary nystagmus

   1. Rapid (10 to 20 beats/second); low amplitude, horizontal eye movements; consists of back-to-back saccades
   2. Patient unable to sustain this type of nystagmus (duration usually less than 30 seconds)
   3. Frequently accompanied by eyelid flutter, convergence, facial grimacing
   4. Can stop nystagmus momentarily by having patient change direction of gaze
   5. Seen in hysterical patients, malingerers (see Chapter 17)

M. Rebound nystagmus

   1. Horizontal jerk nystagmus may be detected as:
      a. Gaze-evoked nystagmus that will slowly fatigue and be followed by development of jerk nystagmus in the opposite direction (ie, fast phase toward the primary position)
      b. Jerk nystagmus that transiently occurs when the eyes are returned to the primary position following sustained eccentric gaze. The nystagmus has its fast phase in the direction opposite to the sustained deviation
   2. Etiologies: brainstem and cerebellar disease

VII. Gaze-evoked nystagmus

A. No nystagmus in primary position of gaze

   1. The specific types of nystagmus described above are generally seen while the eyes are in the primary position
   2. The patients with gaze-evoked nystagmus demonstrate no nystagmus in the primary position and show jerk nystagmus only during eccentric gaze
      a. Left-beating nystagmus on gaze left
      b. Right-beating nystagmus on gaze right
      c. Upbeating nystagmus on gaze up
      d. Downbeating nystagmus on gaze down

B. Downbeating nystagmus seen in gaze down in the patient with gaze-evoked nystagmus does not qualify as and does not have the clinical significance of "downbeat nystagmus" (see Section VI, F, Downbeat nystagmus)

C. The upbeating nystagmus seen in gaze up in the patient with nonspecific, gaze-evoked nystagmus does not qualify as and does not have the clinical significance of "upbeat nystagmus" (see Section VI, G, Upbeat nystagmus)

D. Gaze-evoked nystagmus has two main etiologies:

   1. Drug induced: anticonvulsants (dilantin, phenobarbital) or any kind of tranquilizer or sedative
   2. Posterior fossa disease: bilateral brainstem and/or cerebellar dysfunction (tumor, trauma, demyelination, vascular infarction) involving the neural integrator

E. Gaze-paretic refers to one particular type of gaze-evoked nystagmus, seen in the context of gaze palsy
   1. Slow rate (1 to 2 beats/second)
   2. Large amplitude
   3. Thought to be due to defective gaze-holding mechanism ("leaky" neural integrator)
   4. Patients recovering from a gaze palsy may pass through a stage of gaze-paretic nystagmus

VIII. Saccadic intrusions and oscillations

   A. Saccades are inappropriate if they interfere with foveal fixation of object of interest
   B. Such saccadic intrusions may occur repetitively, causing ocular oscillation
   C. Square-wave jerks
   1. "Fixation instability": nonrhythmic break in fixation followed by a single movement of refoveation
   2. Square-wave jerks are subtle (amplitude, 0.5 to 3.0 degrees; latency to refixation, 200 msec); square-wave pulses are quite easily seen (amplitude, 4 to 30 degrees; latency to refixation, 50 to 150 msec)
   3. So named because of rectangular appearance on eye movement recordings
   4. May occur continuously and then referred to as square-wave oscillations and macro square-wave oscillations
   5. Variety of etiologies including cerebellar disorders, progressive supranuclear palsy, multiple sclerosis, Parkinson's disease
   D. Ocular flutter
   1. Spontaneous intermittent bursts of three or four conjugate back-to-back saccades while the patient is attempting fixation in the primary position
   2. Purely horizontal in direction
   3. No intersaccadic interval as seen with square-wave jerks
   4. Patients with ocular flutter may also demonstrate ocular dysmetria
   E. Opsoclonus
   1. Rapid, involuntary, multivectorial (horizontal, vertical, diagonal), unpredictable (chaotic), conjugate fast eye movements that stop during sleep
   2. Also referred to as "saccadomania"
   3. No intersaccadic intervals
   4. Patients improving from opsoclonus often manifest ocular flutter before recovery
   5. Infants:
        a. Neuroblastoma: opsoclonus is a nonmetastatic, remove effect seen in association with ataxia and myoclonus, and referred to as the syndrome of "dancing eyes and dancing feet"
        b. Infants may also present with opsoclonus that appears due to an autoimmune brainstem encephalitis that is responsive to ACTH
   6. Infants and adults: opsoclonus may be seen as a benign, self-limited ocular phenomenon: a parainfectious encephalopathy
   7. Adults: opsoclonus may be a remote effect of a visceral, lung, breast, or ovarian cancer
   8. Rare causes: toxins, hyperosmolar coma

F. Ocular dysmetria
   1. The ocular equivalent of extremity "past pointing"
   2. Conjugate hypermetric (overshoot) eye movements during voluntary change of gaze
   3. Patients with ocular dysmetria frequently have cerebellar disease and nystagmus on eccentric gaze; therefore, dysmetria is most reliably detected during refixation back to the primary position
   4. During refixation back to the primary position, the eyes will demonstrate their hypermetria, followed by several oscillations about the new fixation point before the eyes come to rest
   5. A single overshoot with corrective saccades is seen at times in the normal subject during small-amplitude saccadic testing

G. Ocular myoclonus
   1. Usually vertical-pendular nystagmus at a rate of two cycles per second
   2. Synchronous contraction of the face, palate, pharynx, diaphragm, extremity may be present
   3. These movements may persist during sleep
   4. Caused by a lesion in the "triangle of Guillain and Mollaret," the triangle connecting the following anatomic sites:
      a. Red nucleus
      b. Ipsilateral inferior olive
      c. Contralateral dentate nucleus
   5. Occurs due to hypertrophy of the inferior olive (latency from acute infarction: 2 to 49 months) and is not a manifestation of acute lesions

H. Ocular bobbing
   1. Fast, conjugate, downward movement of the eye followed by a slow drift back up to the primary position; just like watching a "bobber" on the water as a fish is nibbling at the bait
   2. The patient is usually comatose and has a massive pontine lesion, such as a hemorrhagic, infarct, or malignant tumor
   3. May be seen with obstructive hydrocephalus or metabolic encephalopathy
   4. Usually demonstrates no spontaneous or reflex (doll's eye, calorics) horizontal eye movements

I. Reverse ocular bobbing
   1. Fast, conjugate upward movement followed by slow drift to primary position
   2. Reverse bobbing may occur with metabolic encephalopathy or coexist with ocular bobbing

J. Ocular dipping (inverse bobbing)
   1. Slow, conjugate downward eye movements followed, after variable delay, by quick saccades back to midposition
   2. Etiology: ischemic-hypoxic brainstem insult or metabolic disorder

K. Reverse ocular dipping (converse bobbing)
   1. Slow upward eye movements with rapid return to primary gaze
   2. Etiology: pontine infections, AIDS

L. Superior oblique myokymia
   1. See Chapter 6 (Section VIII)

IX. Periodic deviations

A. Periodic alternating gaze deviation
1. Involuntary, continuous cyclic disorders of eye movements
2. Slow, conjugate deviation of eyes to lateral gaze for about 2 minutes, followed by movement of eyes to opposite lateral gaze position for same time period
3. Continuous cycle but disappears with sleep
4. Seen in alert patients with posterior fossa lesions, hepatic encephalopathy

B. Periodic alternating "ping-pong" gaze
1. Similar to periodic alternating gaze deviation except cycle has periodicity of only a few seconds
2. Comatose patients due to stroke or drug overdose

C. Periodic alternating skew deviation
1. Cyclic alteration of skew deviation over period of 30 seconds to 10 minutes
2. Reported in cases of cerebellar degeneration, and midbrain stroke
3. May occur with periodic alternating nystagmus

X. Special anatomical considerations

A. Acoustic neuroma
1. Slowly growing tumor of the VIII cranial nerve may allow adaptive mechanism to obscure vestibular manifestations
2. Patient may demonstrate peripheral vestibular nystagmus away from the lesion, particularly if fixation is eliminated
3. If tumor expands to compress the brainstem, patient may also develop ipsilateral, slow, large-amplitude, gaze-evoked nystagmus
4. This combination of two nystagmus patterns, termed Bruns' nystagmus, is also seen with other cerebellar-pontine angle masses

B. Lateral medullary (Wallenberg) syndrome
1. Stroke in vascular distribution of posterior-inferior cerebellar artery (PICA)
2. Characteristic neurologic findings:
   a. Dizziness
   b. Ipsilateral limb dysmetria
   c. Ipsilateral impairment of facial sensation
   d. Contralateral dissociated sensory loss
   e. Bulbar impairment
   f. Ipsilateral Horner's syndrome (first-order neuron)
3. Central vestibular nystagmus pattern:
   a. With eyes open, horizontal-torsional jerk nystagmus may beat away from the lesion
   b. With eyes closed, horizontal-torsional jerk nystagmus may beat toward the lesion
4. Lateropulsion of eye and body movements biased toward the side of the lesion
5. Saccadic lateropulsion: all ipsilateral saccades are too large (hypermetric), while those to the opposite side are too small (hypometric)
6. Upward and downward saccades veer ipsilaterally along an oblique rather than vertical line
7. Often accompanied by skew deviation, with the hypotropic eye ipsilateral to the lesion

BIBLIOGRAPHY

Books

Leigh RJ, Zee DS. *The Neurology of Eye Movements.* 3rd ed. New York, NY: Oxford University Press; 1999.

Chapters

Burde RM, Savino PJ, Trobe JD. *Clinical Decisions in Neuro-ophthalmology.* St. Louis, Mo: CV Mosby; 1992: 289-320.

Dell'Osso LF, Daroff RB. Nystagmus and saccadic intrusions and oscillations. In: Duane TD, ed. *Clinical Ophthalmology.* Vol 2. Philadelphia, Pa: Lippincott-Williams & Wilkins; 1997: chapter 11, 1-33.

Fletcher WA. Nystagmus. An overview. In: Sharpe JA, Barber HO, eds. *The Vestibular-Ocular Reflex and Vertigo.* New York, NY: Raven Press; 1993: 195-215.

Leigh, RJ, Averbuch-Heller L. Nystagmus and related motility disorders. In: Miller NR, Newman NJ, eds. *Walsh and Hoyt's Clinical Neuro-ophthalmology.* Vol 1. 5th ed. Baltimore, Md: Williams & Wilkins; 1998: 1461-1505.

Articles

Bosch EP, Kennedy SS, Aschenbrener CA. Ocular bobbing: the myth of its localizing value. *Neurology.* 1975;25:949-953.

Brandt S, Carlsen N, Glentin P, et al. Encephalopathia myoclonica infantalis (Kinsbourne) and neuroblastoma in children. A report of three cases. *Dev Med Child Neurol.* 1974;16:286-294.

Brazis PW. Ocular motor abnormalities in Wallenberg's lateral medullary syndrome. *Mayo Clin Proc.* 1992;67:365-378.

Brusa A, Firpo MP, Massa S, et al. Typical and reverse bobbing. A case with localizing value. *Eur Neurol.* 1984;23:151-155.

Cogan DG. Downbeat nystagmus. *Arch Ophthalmol.* 1968;80:757-768.

Corbett JJ, Schatz NJ, Schults WT, et al. Slowly alternating skew deviation. Description of a pretectal syndrome in there patients. *Ann Neurol.* 1981;10:540-546.

Dell'Osso LF, Schmidt D, Daroff RB. Latent, manifest latent, and congenital nystagmus. *Arch Ophthalmol.* 1979;97:1877-1885.

Dieterich M, Brandt T. Ocular torsion and tilt of subjective visual vertical are sensitive brainstem signs. *Ann Neurol.* 1983;l:292-295.

Digre K. Opsoclonus in adults. Report of three cases and review of the literature. *Arch Neurol.* 1986; 43:1165-1175.

Gottlob I, Wizov SS, Reinecke RD, et al. Spasmus nutans. A long-term follow-up. *Invest Ophthalmology Vis Sci.* 1995;36:2768-2771.

Gottlob I, Zubcov A, Caralano RA, et al. Signs distinguishing spasmus nutans (with and without central nervous system lesions) from infantile nystagmus. *Ophthalmology.* 1990;87:1166-1175.

Hirose G, Kawada J, Tsukada K, et al. Upbeat nystagmus: clinicopathological and pathophysiological considerations. *J Neurol Sci.* 1991;105:159-167.

Kerrison JB, Arnould VJ, Barnada MM, et al. A gene for autosomal dominant congenital nystagmus localizes to 6p12. *Genomics.* 1996;33:523-526.

Lopez LI, Gresty MA, Bronstein AM, et al. Acquired pendular nystagmus; oculomotor and MRI findings. *Brain*. 1996;119:265-272.

Masucci EF, Fabara JA, Saini N, et al. Periodic alternating ping-pong gaze. *Arch Ophthalmol*. 1981; 131:1123-1127.

Stewart JD, Kirkham THE, Mathieson G. Periodic alternating gaze. *Neurology*. 1979;29:222-224.

Susac JO, Hoyt WE, Daroff RB, et al. Clinical spectrum of ocular bobbing. *J Neurol Neurosurg Psychiatry*. 1970;33:771-775.

Van Weerden TW, Van Woerkom TCAM. Ocular dipping. *Clin Neurol Neurosurg*. 1982;84:221-226.

Yee RD. Downbeat nystagmus: characteristics and localization of lesions. *Trans Am Ophthalmol Soc*. 1989;87:948-1032.

Zahn JR. Incidence and characteristics of voluntary nystagmus. *J Neurol Neurosurg Psychiatry*. 1978; 41:617-618.

Chapter 4

The Six Syndromes of the VI Nerve (Abducens)

I. Anatomical considerations

A. Figure 4-1a identifies the structures in the posterior fossa, base of the skull, and middle cranial fossa that serve as landmarks in the study of the VI nerve

B. Figure 4-2 is a schematic representation of these structures and includes a sagittal section of the brainstem

C. Figure 4-3 is a schematic representation of these structures when viewed from the occipital pole

D. Figure 4-4 illustrates the S-shaped course of the VI nerve and shows its relationship to the VII and VIII cranial nerves and the internal carotid artery

E. Figure 4-5 adds the III, IV, and V cranial nerves

F. Figure 4-6 shows the composite diagram and the division of the course of the VI nerve into five portions, each associated with a different syndrome:
1. VI^1: The brainstem syndrome
2. VI^2: The subarachnoid space syndrome
3. VI^3: The petrous apex syndrome
4. VI^4: The cavernous sinus syndrome
5. VI^5: The orbital syndrome

II. The brainstem syndrome (VI^1)

A. Figure 4-6 reminds us that a brainstem lesion of the VI nerve may also affect V, VII, VIII nerves and the cerebellum

B. The VI nerve nucleus contains motoneurons that supply the lateral rectus muscle and abducens internuclear neurons that project via the medial longitudinal fasciculus (MLF) to the medial rectus subdivision of the contralateral oculomotor nucleus. Thus, a nuclear VI nerve palsy causes an ipsilateral conjugate horizontal gaze palsy

C. Figure 4-7 illustrates the structures within the substance of the lower pons that may be affected by a lesion affecting the VI nerve
1. Oculosympathetic central neuron: ipsilateral Horner's syndrome

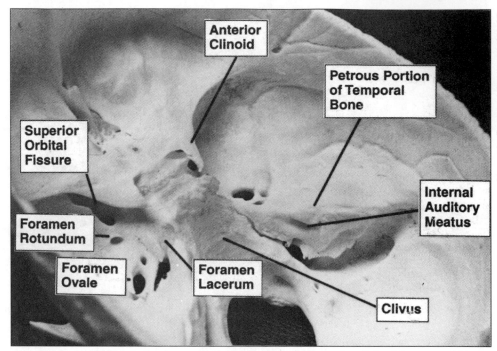

Figure 4-1a. Human skull. Anatomical landmarks in the study of the VI nerve. Oblique superotemporal view.

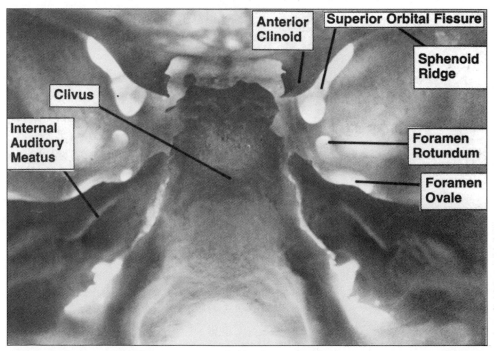

Figure 4-1b. Human skull. Anatomical landmarks in the study of the VI nerve. Occipital view, retroilluminated skull.

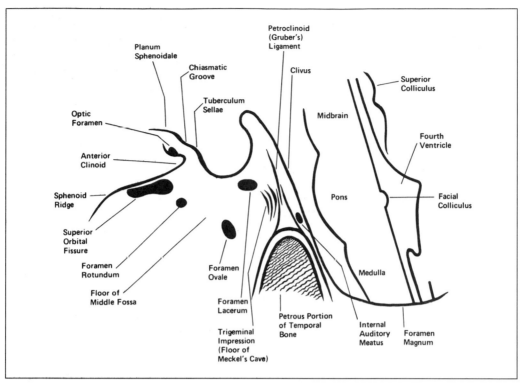

Figure 4-2. Schematic representation of the landmarks, temporal view.

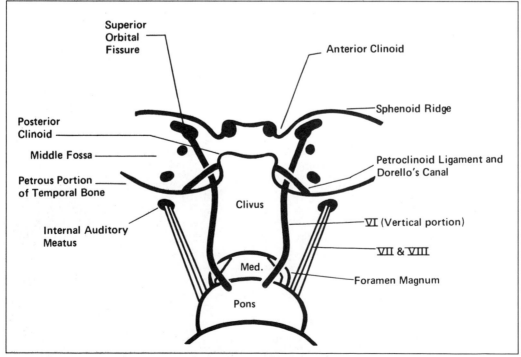

Figure 4-3. Schematic representation of the anatomical landmarks, occipital view.

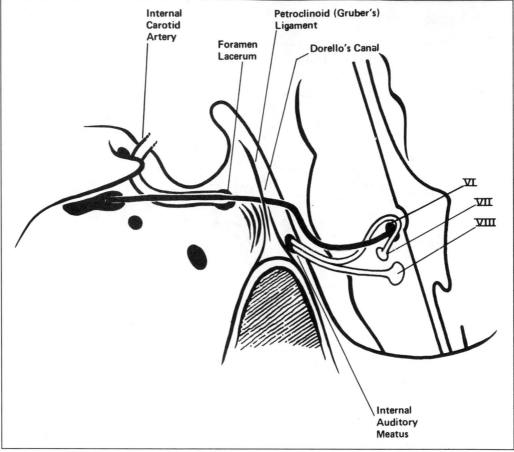

Figure 4-4. Course of the VI nerve (highlighted in black) from the pons to the superior orbital tissue.

      2. PPRF: ipsilateral horizontal conjugate gaze palsy

      3. MLF: ipsilateral internuclear ophthalmoplegia

      4. Pyramidal tract: contralateral hemiparesis

  D. The brainstem syndrome may consist of any combination of the deficits listed above; the following are frequently encountered syndromes:

      1. Millard-Gubler syndrome

         a. VI nerve paresis

         b. Ipsilateral VII nerve paresis

         c. Contralateral hemiparesis

      2. Raymond's syndrome

         a. VI nerve paresis

         b. Contralateral hemiparesis

      3. Foville's syndrome

         a. Horizontal conjugate gaze palsy

         b. Ipsilateral V, VII, VIII cranial nerve palsies

         c. Ipsilateral Horner's syndrome

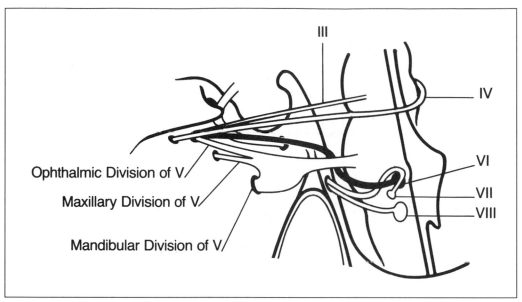

Figure 4-5. Composite diagram illustrating the III through VIII cranial nerves.

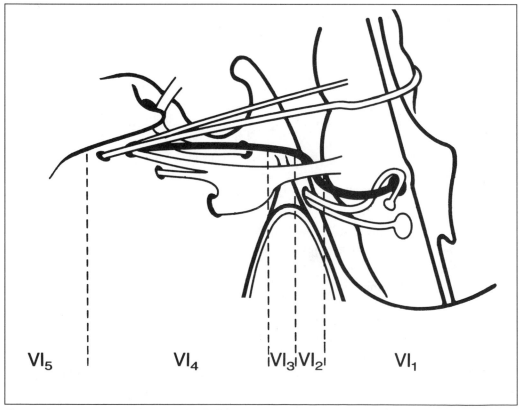

Figure 4-6. Composite diagram divided into five sections, corresponding to the first five syndromes of the VI nerve (VI^1 to VI^5).

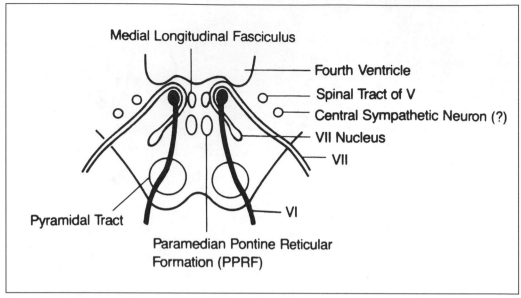

Figure 4-7. Diagram of cross-section of the lower pons through the VI nucleus and fascile (high-lighted in black).

III. The subarachnoid space syndrome (VI²)

A. Elevated intracranial pressure (ICP) may result in downward displacement of the brain-stem, with stretching of the VI nerve, which is tethered at its exit from the pons and in Dorello's canal

1. Gives rise to "nonlocalizing" VI nerve palsies of raised ICP
2. Approximately 30% of patients with pseudotumor cerebri have VI nerve paresis, the only neurologic deficit they are allowed, besides papilledema and its visual field changes

B. Other disturbances in the subarachnoid space causing VI nerve palsies include hemor-rhage, meningeal or parameningeal infection (eg, viral, bacterial, fungal), inflammation (eg, sarcoidosis), or infiltration (eg, lymphoma, leukemia, carcinoma)

IV. The petrous apex syndrome (VI³)

A. Contact with the tip of the petrous pyramid makes the portion of the VI nerve within Dorello's canal susceptible to pathologic processes affecting the petrous bone

B. Gradenigo's syndrome

1. Clinical findings
   a. VI nerve palsy
   b. Ipsilateral decreased hearing
   c. Ipsilateral facial pain in the distribution of the V nerve
   d. Ipsilateral facial paralysis
2. Due to localized inflammation or extradural abscess of petrous apex following com-plicated otitis media

C. Petrous bone fracture
  1. Basal skull fracture following head trauma
  2. Potential cranial nerve involvement: V, VI, VII, VIII
  3. Associated findings: hemotympanum, Battle's sign, mastoid ecchymosis, CSF otor-rhea

D. Pseudo-Gradenigo's syndrome
  1. Nasopharyngeal carcinoma may cause serous otitis media due to obstruction of the eustachian tube and the carcinoma may subsequently invade the cavernous sinus, causing VI nerve paresis
  2. Cerebellopontine angle tumor: may cause VI nerve paresis and other clinical findings, including:
    a. Decreased hearing
    b. VII nerve palsy
    c. V nerve paralysis
    d. Ataxia
    e. Papilledema

V. The cavernous sinus syndrome (VI^4)

A. Lesions in cavernous sinus rarely produce isolated VI nerve palsy; associated involvement of:
  1. III, IV, and ophthalmic (V^l) nerves
  2. Carotid oculosympathetic plexus (Horner's syndrome)
  3. Optic nerve and chiasm
  4. Pituitary gland

B. Differential diagnosis of cavernous sinus disease includes:
  1. Trauma
  2. Vascular
  3. Neoplastic
  4. Inflammatory

C. See Chapter 7

VI. The orbital syndrome (VI^5)

A. Proptosis is an early sign and may be accompanied by congestion of the conjunctival vessels and chemosis

B. The optic nerve may appear normal or demonstrate atrophy or edema

C. Trigeminal signs are limited to the ophthalmic division

D. It is frequently difficult to distinguish between cranial nerve (III, IV, VI) pareses and mechanical restriction of the globe

E. Etiologies
  1. Tumor (local, metastatic)
  2. Trauma
  3. Inflammatory pseudotumor
  4. Cellulitis

Table 4-1

ETIOLOGIES OF ACQUIRED VI NERVE PALSY

	Rucker (1958)	Schrader (1960) (Isolated VI)	Rucker (1966)	Johnston (1968)	Robertson (1970) (Children)	Rush (1981)	Kodsi (1992) (Children)	Richards (1992)
Total # Patients	545	104	607	158	133	419	88	575
Etiologies (%)								
Neoplasm	21	7	33	13	39	15	21	20
Trauma	16	3	12	32	20	17	42	20
Aneurysm	6	0	3	1	3	3	0	3
Ischemic	11	36	8	16	0	18	0	10
Miscellaneous	16	30	24	30	29	18	22	23
Undetermined	30	24	20	8	9	29	15	23

VII. Isolated VI nerve palsy (VI[6])

  A. The sixth syndrome of the VI nerve

      1. No signs of the first five syndromes

      2. Frequently seen as a postviral syndrome in young patients and as an ischemic mononeuropathy in adults

      3. As a general rule:

          a. Ocular motor cranial nerve palsy in young patient—greater likelihood of neoplasm; aggressive workup

          b. Ocular motor cranial nerve palsy in older patient—greater likelihood of ischemic mononeuropathy; less aggressive workup

      4. Note in series by Robertson and Kodsi (Table 4-1) that if cases due to trauma are excluded, a child with a VI nerve palsy has a 50-50 chance of harboring a neoplasm, usually a brainstem glioma

  B. Initial evaluation

      1. Blood pressure determination

      2. Blood tests

          a. Complete blood count (CBC)

          b. Glucose tolerance test (GTT)

          c. Sedimentation rate

          d. VDRL and FTA-ABS (or TPHA)

          e. ANA (antinuclear antibody)

      3. Radiographic studies

          a. Patients under age 40 should undergo cranial magnetic resonance (MR) scanning

          b. In patients less than 15 years old, a postviral syndrome must be kept in mind. It will follow a benign course and completely resolve in 4 months

          c. In patients over age 40, the most likely cause is an ischemic mononeuropathy. If the VI nerve palsy has not resolved in 4 months, or if other cranial nerve involvement occurs, then comprehensive evaluation is recommend

    i. Medical and neurologic examinations

    ii. CT scan

    iii. Magnetic resonance imaging (MRI)

    iv. Lumbar puncture

    v. Cerebral angiography

VIII. Table 4-1 contains a summary of eight retrospective studies of patients with paresis of the VI nerve

A. Eight to 30%, etiology undetermined, reflecting the vulnerability of the nerve to influences that are transient, benign, and unrecognizable

B. Sixteen to 30% attributed to a miscellaneous group of causes that includes leukemia, migraine, pseudotumor cerebri, multiple sclerosis, myelography. The miscellaneous group of etiologies reflects the poor localizing value of paresis of the VI nerve

IX. The six impostors of the VI nerve

A. Thyroid eye disease

B. Myasthenia gravis

C. Duane's syndrome

D. Spasm of the near reflex

E. Medial wall orbital blowout fracture with restrictive myopathy

F. Break in fusion of a congenital esophoria

BIBLIOGRAPHY

Chapters

Glover JS, Siatkowski RM. Infranuclear disorders of eye movements. In: Duane TD, ed. *Clinical Ophthalmology.* Vol 2. Philadelphia, Pa: Lippincott-William & Wilkins; 1998: chapter 12, 1-63.

Leigh RJ, Zee DS. *The Neurology of Eye Movements.* 3rd ed. New York, NY: Oxford University Press; 1999: 321-404.

Smith C. Nuclear and and infranuclear ocular motility disorders. In: Miller NR, Newman NJ, eds. *Walsh and Hoyt's Clinical Neuro-ophthalmology.* 5th ed. Vol 1. Baltimore, Md: Williams & Wilkins; 1998: 1189-1281.

Articles

Duane A. Congenital deficiency of abduction associated with impairment of adduction, retraction movements, contraction of the palpebral fissure, and oblique movements of the eye. *Arch Ophthalmol.* 1905;34:133-159.

Galetta SL, Smith JL. Chronic isolated sixth nerve palsies. *Arch Neurol.* 1989,46:79-82.

Godtfredsen E, Lederman M. Diagnostic and prognostic roles of ophthalmic neurologic signs and symptoms in malignant nasopharyngeal tumors. *Am J Ophthalmol.* 1965;59:1063-1069.

Gradenigo G. A special syndrome of endocranial otitic complications (paralysis of the motor oculi externus of otitic origin). *Ann Otol.* 1904;13:637.

Hotchkiss MG, Miller NR, Clark AW, et al. Bilateral Duane's retraction syndrome. A clinical pathologic case report. *Arch Ophthalmol.* 1980;98:870-874.

Jacobson DM. Progressive ophthalmoplegia with acute ischemic abducens palsies. *Am J Ophthalmol.* 1996;122:278-279.

Johnston AC. Etiology and treatment of abducens palsy. *Trans Pac Coast Oto-ophthalmol Soc.* 1968;49:259-277.

Knox D, Clark D, Schuster F. Benign VI nerve palsies in children. *Pediatrics.* 1967;40:560-564.

Kodsi SR, Younge BR. Acquired oculomotor, trochlear, abducent cranial nerve palsies in pediatric patients. *Am J Ophthalmol.* 1992;114:568-574.

Moster ML, Savino PJ, Sergott RC, et al. Isolated sixth nerve palsies in younger adults. *Arch Ophthalmol.* 1984;102:1328-1330.

Richards BW, Jones FR, Young BR. Causes and prognosis in 4278 cases of paralysis of the oculomotor, trochlear, and abducens cranial nerves. *Am J Ophthalmol.* 1992;113:489-496.

Robertson DM, Hines JD, Rucker CW. Acquired sixth nerve paresis in children. *Arch Ophthalmol.* 1970;83:574-579.

Rucker CW. Paralysis of the third, fourth, and sixth cranial nerves. *Am J Ophthalmol.* 1958;46:787-794.

Rucker CW. The causes of paralysis of the third, fourth, and sixth cranial nerves. *Am J Ophthalmol.* 1966;61:1293-1298.

Rush JA, Younge BR. Paralysis of cranial nerves III, IV and VI. Cause and prognosis in 1,000 cases. *Arch Ophthalmol.* 1981;99:76-79.

Sakalas R, Harbison JW, Vines FS, Becker DP. Chronic sixth nerve palsy. An initial sign of basisphenoid tumors. *Arch Ophthalmol.* 1975;93:186-190.

Savino PJ, Hilliker JK, Cassell GH, et al. Chronic sixth nerve palsies. *Arch Ophthalmol.* 1982;100:1442-1444.

Volpe NJ, Lessell S. Remitting sixth nerve palsy in skull base tumors. *Arch Ophthamol.* 1993;111:1391-1395.

Chapter 5

The Seven Syndromes of the III Nerve (Oculomotor)

I. Anatomical considerations

A. Figure 5-1 represents a cross-section through the rostral midbrain at the level of the superior colliculi

B. Figure 5-2 is a copy of Figure 5-1 with superimposition of sites 1 through 6, representing six sites in which the III cranial nerve may be affected and present with distinct ocular manifestations, or in the company of different neurologic signs and symptoms, or as a result of specific disease processes. The seventh syndrome is the isolated III nerve palsy

C. Figure 5-3 illustrates the relationship of the III nerve (highlighted in black) to other cranial nerves

II. The seven syndromes of the III nerve

A. Nuclear III nerve paresis (see Figure 5-2, site 1)

    1. Extremely rare

    2. The arrangement of the III nerve subnuclei places strict prerequisites on the diagnosis of a nuclear III nerve palsy

        a. Each superior rectus is innervated by the contralateral III nerve nucleus; therefore, a nuclear III nerve palsy on one side requires paresis of the contralateral superior rectus

        b. Both levators are innervated by one subnuclear structure—the central caudal nucleus; therefore, a nuclear III nerve palsy requires bilateral ptosis

    3. Some cases of skew deviation may actually represent instances of one or more III nerve subnuclei (subserving the vertical recti or the inferior oblique) being affected

B. III nerve fascicle syndrome (see Figure 5-2, site 2)

    1. Topical diagnosis depends upon the coexistence of other neurologic signs

    2. Fascicles have already left the III nerve nucleus so that the ocular manifestations are present only on one side (no longer subject to the rules governing nuclear III nerve paresis)

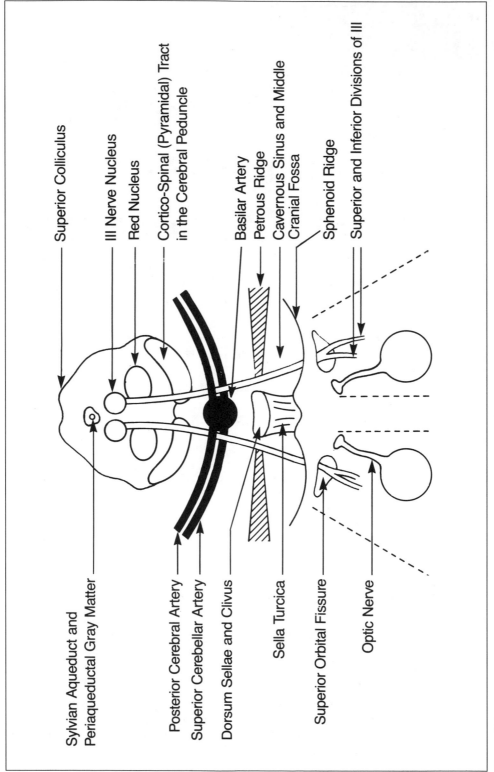

Superior Colliculus

III Nerve Nucleus

Red Nucleus

Cortico-Spinal (Pyramidal) Tract
in the Cerebral Peduncle

Basilar Artery

Petrous Ridge

Cavernous Sinus and Middle
Cranial Fossa

Sphenoid Ridge

Superior and Inferior Divisions of III

Sylvian Aqueduct and
Periaqueductal Gray Matter

Posterior Cerebral Artery

Superior Cerebellar Artery

Dorsum Sellae and Clivus

Sella Turcica

Superior Orbital Fissure

Optic Nerve

Figure 5-1.

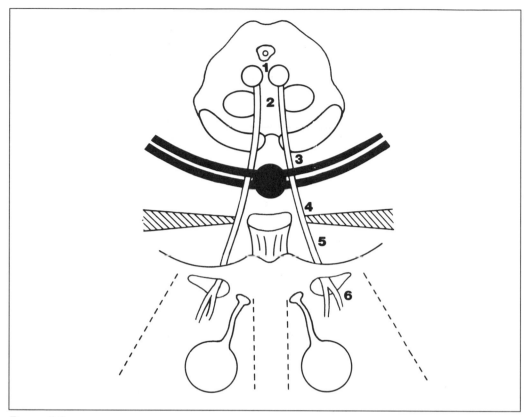

Figure 5-2.

        3. Nothnagel's syndrome
            a. Lesion in the area of the superior cerebellar peduncle
            b. Ipsilateral III nerve paresis and cerebellar ataxia
        4. Benedikt's syndrome
            a. Lesion in the region of the red nucleus
            b. Ipsilateral III nerve paresis with contralateral hemitremor
        5. Weber's syndrome
            a. Involvement of the III nerve in the neighborhood of the cerebral peduncle
            b. Ipsilateral III nerve paresis with contralateral hemiparesis
        6. Claude's syndrome
            a. Features of both Benedikt's and Nothnagel's syndromes
        7. Fascicular lesions are virtually always ischemic, infiltrative (tumor), or rarely inflammatory
    C. Uncal hemiation syndrome (see Figure 5-2, site 3)
        1. In its course toward the cavernous sinus, the III nerve rests on the edge of the tentorium cerebelli
        2. The portion of the brain overlying the III nerve, at the tentorial edge, is the uncal portion of the undersurface of the temporal lobe

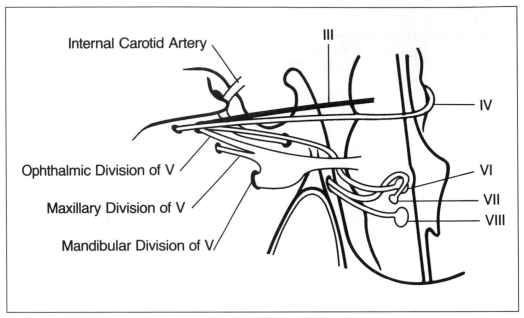

Figure 5-3.

    3. A supratentorial space-occupying mass, located anywhere in or above this cerebral hemisphere, may cause a downward displacement and herniation of the uncus across the tentorial edge, thereby compressing the III nerve (Figure 5-4)

    4. A dilated and fixed pupil (Hutchinson pupil) may be the first indication that altered consciousness is due to a space-occupying intracranial lesion

  D. Posterior communicating artery aneurysm (see Figure 5-2, site 4)

    1. In its course toward the cavernous sinus, the III nerve travels alongside (lateral to) the posterior communicating artery

    2. The most common cause of nontraumatic isolated III nerve paresis with pupillary involvement is an aneurysm at the junction of the posterior communicating artery and the internal carotid artery (Figure 5-5)

    3. Hemorrhage suddenly enlarges the aneurysmal sac to which the III nerve is adherent or there is actual hemorrhage into the substance of the nerve

    4. On occasion, the pupil is spared early in the course of aneurysmal compression of the III nerve. The patient must be followed carefully during the initial 5 to 7 days to be certain of the status of the pupil

  E. Cavernous sinus syndrome (see Figure 5-2, site 5)

    1. III nerve paresis is usually seen in association with other cranial nerve involvement: IV, V, VI, and oculosympathetic paralysis

    2. III nerve paresis due to cavernous sinus lesion tends to be partial (ie, all muscles innervated by the III nerve are not equally involved)

    3. Pupillary fibers are frequently "spared," such that the pupil may be normal or minimally involved

    4. Cavernous sinus lesions may lead to primary aberrant regeneration of the III nerve (see below)

    5. See Chapter 7

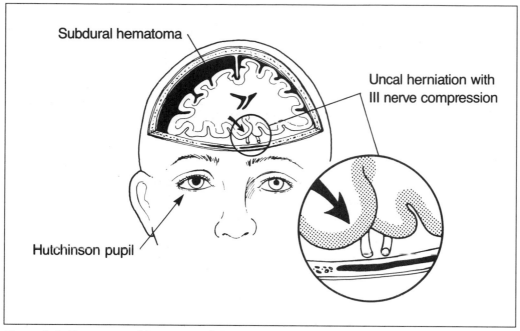

Figure 5-4. Transtentorial herniation of the uncus with III nerve compression.

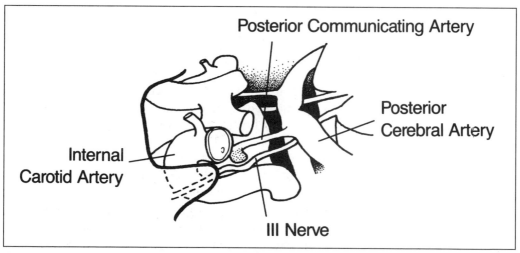

Figure 5-5. Compression of the left III nerve due to aneurysm at the junction of the posterior communicating and internal carotid arteries.

F. Orbital syndrome (see Figure 5-2, site 6)
    1. See the orbital syndrome of the VI nerve (Chapter 4)
    2. Just before entering the superior orbital fissure, the III nerve splits into two divisions
    3. The superior division innervates the:
        a. Superior rectus
        b. Levator palpebrae

4. The inferior division innervates the:
   a. Inferior rectus
   b. Medial rectus
   c. Inferior oblique
   d. Pupil (iris sphincter muscle)
   e. Accommodation (ciliary muscle)
5. Orbital involvement of the III nerve may result in selective paresis of structures innervated by only one of the divisions

G. Pupil-sparing isolated III nerve paresis (the seventh syndrome of the III nerve)
   1. The pupillomotor fibers of the III nerve travel in the outer layers of the nerve and are therefore closer to the nutrient blood supply enveloping the nerve
   2. This may explain why the pupillomotor fibers are spared in 80% of ischemic III nerve pareses but are affected in 95% of cases of compressive (trauma, tumor, aneurysm) III nerve paresis
   3. Patients with pupil-sparing isolated III nerve palsies are evaluated and managed in a similar manner to patients with isolated IV and VI nerve pareses
      a. Ischemia lab workup
         i. Blood pressure determination
         ii. Complete blood count (CBC)
         iii. Sedimentation rate
         iv. Glucose tolerance test
         v. VDRL and FTA-ABS (or TPHA)
         vi. ANA (antinuclear antibody)
      b. Follow the patient for 3 to 4 months if:
         i. The III nerve paresis is truly isolated
         ii. The patient is over 40 years of age
         iii. The patient has a history of diabetes or hypertension
      c. Most patients with ischemic III nerve paresis demonstrate improvement of the motility measurements within 1 month and may have complete recovery by 3 months (maximum: 6 months)
      d. Recommend cranial magnetic resonance (MR) scanning, MR angiography, lumbar puncture, and four-vessel cerebral angiography if:
         i. The pupil becomes dilated in the initial 5 to 7 days after onset
         ii. No significant improvement in 3 months
         iii. The patient develops signs of aberrant regeneration of the III nerve
         iv. Other neurologic findings develop
      e. **Caution:** ocular myasthenia can mimic a pupil-sparing III nerve palsy; remember the Tensilon test!

III. **Incidence of various causes of III nerve palsies**
   A. Table 5-1 summarizes seven major published series of patients with paresis of the oculomotor nerve
   B. Although neoplasm, aneurysm, and ischemia are the most common etiologies, approximately 10% to 25% of cases of III nerve palsies have an undetermined cause

Table 5-1

ETIOLOGIES OF ACQUIRED III NERVE PALSY

	Rucker (1958)	Goldstein (1960) (Isolated III)	Green (1966)	Rucker (1966)	Rush (1981)	Kodsi (1992) (Children)	Richards (1992)
Total # Patients	335	61	130	274	290	35	244
Etiologies (%)							
Neoplasm	11	10	4	18	12	14	10
Trauma	15	8	11	13	16	40	14
Aneurysm	19	18	30	18	14	0	12
Ischemic*	19	47	19	17	21	0	23
Miscellaneous	8	6	13	12	14	29	18
Undetermined	28	11	23	20	23	17	23

*Including diabetes mellitus

C. Approximately one-half of III nerve palsies in children are congenital and a high percentage have signs of aberrant regeneration. However, approximately 10% to 20% are due to aneurysm or neoplasm; therefore, all children should undergo MR scanning

IV. **Aberrant regeneration (misdirection) of the III nerve**

  A. Regeneration of the disrupted III nerve fibers may result in fibers of one structure being hooked up ("axon sprouting") to fibers that terminate in another structure

  B. Clinical phenomena may be classified as:

   1. Lid-gaze dyskinesis

     a. Some of the inferior rectus fibers may end up innervating the levator so that the lid retracts when the patient looks down: pseudo-von Graefe's sign

     b. Some of the medial rectus fibers may end up supplying some of the innervation to the levator so that the lid retracts when the patient adducts his or her eye: inverse Duane's syndrome

   2. Pupil-gaze dyskinesis

     a. Some of the medial rectus fibers may end up innervating the pupillary sphincter muscle so that there is more pupil constriction during convergence than as a response to light: pseudo-Argyll Robertson pupil

     b. Some of the fibers destined to innervate the inferior rectus may end up innervating the pupillary sphincter so that on attempted downgaze, the pupil constricts

  C. Two forms of aberrant regeneration are:

   1. Primary aberrant regeneration

     a. No preceding acute III nerve palsy

     b. Insidious development of III nerve palsy with accompanying signs of misdirection

     c. Sign of an intracavernous lesion: meningioma, aneurysm, neurinoma

   2. Secondary aberrant regeneration

a. Observe weeks to months during recovery from a III nerve palsy

b. Seen after trauma and tumor compression of the III nerve, but never after ischemic III nerve paresis. If you are following a patient with a presumed diagnosis of ischemic III nerve palsy and he or she develops signs of aberrant regeneration, then MR scanning and cerebral angiography are indicated

V. Rare causes of III nerve palsy

A. Minor head trauma

1. In general, head trauma causing III nerve palsy is severe enough to cause loss of consciousness and often other neurologic deficits
2. Rarely, a patient may harbor a basal intracranial tumor and, with only minor head trauma, develop a III nerve palsy
3. Minimal head injury resulting in a III nerve palsy is an indication for cranial MR scanning

B. Ophthalmoplegic migraine

1. Onset almost always in childhood
2. Usually a family history of migraine
3. III nerve palsy may occur at any time in relation to headache but usually appears as the headache phase abates
4. As a rule, III nerve palsy clears completely within 1 month, but occasionally permanent oculomotor paresis occurs

C. Cyclic oculomotor palsy

1. Disorder usually present at birth or in early childhood
2. Occurs in the setting of a total III nerve palsy
3. Spastic movements of the muscles innervated by the III nerve results in lid elevation, adduction, miosis, and increased accommodation
4. These movements occur at regular intervals, lasting 10 to 30 seconds
5. Etiology unknown

BIBLIOGRAPHY

Chapters

Glaser JS, Siatkowski RM. Infranuclear disorders of eye movements. In: Duane TD, ed. *Duane's Clinical Ophthalmology.* Vol 2. Philadelphia, Pa: Lippincott-Williams & Wilkins; 1998: chapter 12, 1-63.

Leigh RJ, Zee DS. *The Neurology of Eye Movements.* 3rd ed. New York, NY: Oxford University Press; 1999: 321-404.

Smith C. Nuclear and infranuclear ocular motility disorders. In: Miller NR, Newman NJ, eds. *Walsh and Hoyt's Clinical Neuro-ophthalmology.* 5th ed. Vol 1. Baltimore, Md: Williams & Wilkins; 1998: 1189-1281.

Articles

Asbury AK, Aldredge H, Hirshberg R, et al. Oculomotor palsy in diabetes mellitus: a clinicopathological study. *Brain.* 1970;93:555-566.

Brazis PW. Localization of lesions of the oculomotor nerve: recent concepts. *Mayo Clin Proc.* 1991; 66:1029-1035.

Cox TA, Wurster IB, Godfrey WA. Primary aberrant oculomotor regeneration due to intracranial aneurysm. *Arch Neurol.* 1979;36:570-571.

Eyster EF, Hoyt WF, Wilson CB. Oculomotor palsy from minor head trauma. An initial sign of basal intracranial tumor. *JAMA.* 1972;220:1083-1086.

Friedman AP, Harter DH, Merritt HH. Ophthalmoplegic migraine. *Arch Neurol.* 1962;7:320-327.

Goldstein JE, Cogan DG. Diabetic ophthalmoplegia with special reference to the pupil. *Arch Ophthalmol.* 1960;64:592-600.

Harley RD. Paralytic strabismus in children: etiologic incidence and management of the third, fourth, and sixth nerve palsies. *Ophthalmology.* 1980;87:24-43.

Hopf HC, Gutman L. Diabetic third nerve palsy: evidence for a mesencephalic lesion. *Neurology.* 1990;40:1041-1045.

Jacobson DM. Pupil involvement in patients with diabetes-associated oculomotor nerve palsy. *Arch Ophthalmol.* 1998;116:723-727.

Jacobson DM, Broste SK. Early progression of ophthalmoplegia in patients with ischemic oculomotor nerve palsies. *Arch Ophthalmol.* 1995;113:1525-1537.

Jacobson DM, Trobe JD. The emerging role of magnetic resonance imaging in the management of patients with third cranial nerve palsy. *Am J Ophthalmol.* 1999;128:94-96.

Kerr FWL, Hollowell OW. Location of pupillomotor and accommodation fibers in the oculomotor nerve: experimental observation in paralytic mydriasis. *J Neurol Neurosurg Psychiatry.* 1964;27:473-481.

Kissel JT, Burde RM, Klingele TG, et al. Pupil-sparing oculomotor palsies with internal carotid-posterior communicating artery aneurysms. *Ann Neurol.* 1983;13:149-154.

Kodsi SR, Younge BR. Acquired oculomotor, trochlear and abducent cranial nerve palsies in pediatric patients. *Am J Ophthalmol.* 1992;114:568-574.

Lepore FE, Glaser JS. Misdirection revisited: a critical appraisal of acquired oculomotor nerve synkinesis. *Arch Ophthamol.* 1980;98:2206-2209.

Loewenfeld IE, Thompson HS. Oculomotor paresis with cyclical spasms. A critical review of the literature and a new case. *Arch Ophthalmol.* 1975;20:81-124.

Miller NR. Solitary oculomotor nerve palsy in childhood. *Am J Ophthalmol.* 1977;83:106-111.

Richards BW, Jones FR, Younge BR. Causes and prognosis in 4278 cases of paralysis of the oculomotor, trochlear and abducens cranial nerves. *Am J Ophthalmol.* 1992;113:489-496.

Rucker CW. Paralysis of the third, fourth, and sixth cranial nerves. *Am J Ophthalmol.* 1958;46:787-794.

Rucker CW. The causes of paralysis of the third, fourth, and sixth cranial nerves. *Am J Ophthalmol.* 1966;61:1293-1298.

Rush JA, Younge BR. Paralysis of cranial nerves III, IV, and VI. Cause and prognosis in 1,000 cases. *Arch Ophthalmol.* 1981;99:76-79.

Schatz NJ, Savino PJ, Corbett JJ. Primary aberrant oculomotor regeneration. A sign of intracavernous meningioma. *Arch Neurol.* 1977;34:29-32.

Warwick R. Representation of the extraocular muscles in the oculomotor nuclei of the monkey. *J Comp Neurol.* 1953;98:449-495.

Weber RB, Daroff RB, Mackey EM. Pathology of oculomotor nerve palsy in diabetics. *Neurology.* 1970;20:835-838.

Chapter 6

The Five Syndromes of the IV Nerve (Trochlear)

I. **Anatomical considerations**

A. Figure 6-1 is a diagram of a cross-section of the lower midbrain at the level of the inferior colliculi

B. The IV nerve is:
1. The only cranial nerve that exits at the dorsal aspect of the brainstem (Figure 6-2)
2. The cranial nerve with the longest intracranial course (75 mm)

C. The IV nerve fascicles cross in the anterior medullary velum (roof of the Sylvian Aqueduct) prior to exiting dorsally and coursing anteriorly around the midbrain to travel forward between the superior cerebellar and posterior cerebral arteries (just as, but laterally separated from, the III cranial nerve)

D. Therefore, the left IV nerve fascicle becomes the right IV nerve and innervates the right superior oblique muscle; and the right IV nerve fascicle becomes the left IV nerve and innervates the left superior oblique muscle

II. **Clinical syndromes of the IV nerve (Figure 6-3): nuclear-fascicular syndrome, subarachnoid space syndrome, cavernous sinus syndrome, orbital syndrome, isolated IV nerve palsy (congenital or acquired)**

A. Nuclear-fascicular syndrome (see Figure 6-3, site 1)
1. Distinguishing nuclear from fascicular lesions is virtually impossible due to the short course of the fascicles within the midbrain, thus the lack of associated neurologic signs
2. Frequent etiologies include hemorrhage, infarction, demyelination, trauma (including neurosurgical)
3. Fascicular lesion may be seen with contralateral Horner's syndrome, since the sympathetic pathways descend through the dorsolateral tegmentum of the midbrain adjacent to the trochlear fascicles

B. Subarachnoid space syndrome (see Figure 6-3, site 2)
1. IV nerve particularly susceptible to injury as it emerges from the dorsal surface of brainstem

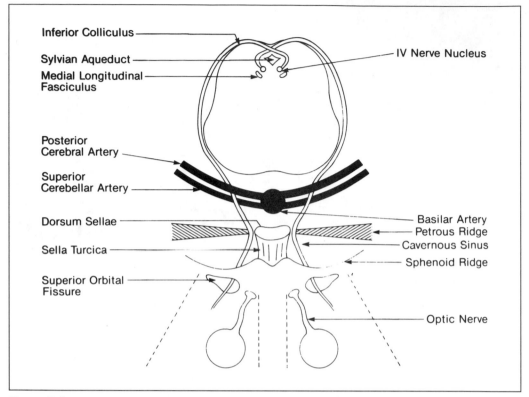

Figure 6-1.

2. When bilateral IV nerve palsies occur, the site of injury is likely in the anterior medullary velum. Contrecoup forces transmitted to the brainstem by the free tentorial edge may injure the nerves at this site

3. Less frequent causes include tumor (eg, pinealoma, tentorial meningioma), meningitis, neurosurgical trauma

C. Cavernous sinus syndrome (see Figure 6-3, site 3)

1. Seen in association with other cranial nerve palsies: III, V, VI oculosympathetic paralysis

2. Checking IV nerve function in the setting of a III nerve paresis

a. Since the involved eye cannot be adducted well, the vertical actions of the superior oblique muscle cannot be tested

b. Therefore, the eye is moved into abduction and then the patient is instructed to look down; the ability of the eye to intort is examined as a measure of IV nerve function

c. If a limbal or conjunctival landmark (eg, pterygium or blood vessel) is noted to intort, then the IV nerve is presumed intact

3. See Chapter 7

D. Orbital syndrome (see Figure 6-3, site 4)

1. Usually seen in association with III, IV, and VI cranial nerve palsies: orbital signs including proptosis, chemosis, conjunctival injection

2. Major etiologies include trauma, inflammation, tumor

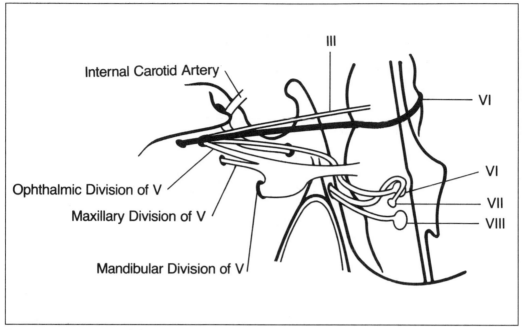

Figure 6-2. Diagram of the IV nerve (highlighted in black) and its relationship to cranial nerves III through VIII.

E. Isolated IV nerve palsy (the fifth syndrome of the IV nerve)
  1. Congenital
      a. See Section VI for incidence of this condition
      b. Most often seen in pediatric population and late in life (fifth to seventh decades) as patient's IV nerve palsy may decompensate
      c. Diagnostic keys
          i. Large vertical fusion amplitude (10 to 15 prism diopters)
          ii. FAT (family album tomography) scan: look at old photographs to detect long-standing head tilt, indicative of congenital etiology
  2. Acquired
      a. Acute onset of vertical diplopia, usually with torsional component
      b. Characteristic head position
          i. Tilt to opposite shoulder
          ii. Head turned downward with chin depressed, eyes up
          iii. Face turned to opposite side
      c. Must perform Parks-Bielschowsky three-step test (see below) to confirm diagnosis
      d. Initial evaluation
          i. Blood pressure determination
          ii. Glucose tolerance test (GTT)
          iii. Sedimentation rate
      e. As with other isolated ocular motor neuropathies, if the IV nerve palsy has not improved or resolved within 4 months, or if other neurologic signs develop, further workup is indicated

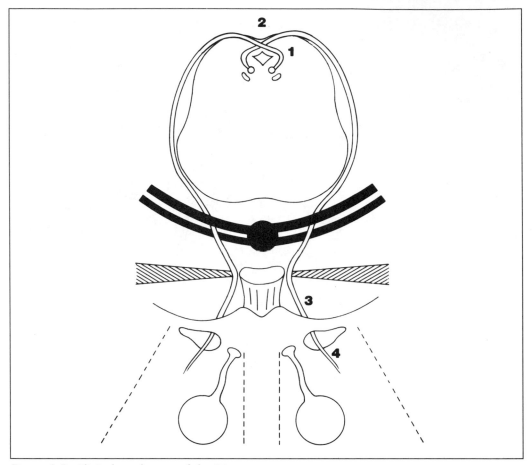

Figure 6-3. Clinical syndromes of the IV nerve.

> i. Medical and neurologic examinations
> ii. Computed tomographic (CT) scanning
> iii. Magnetic resonance (MR) scanning
> iv. Lumbar puncture
> v. Cerebral angiography

III. Diagnosis of recently acquired IV nerve palsy

A. If a patient has vertical misalignment (hypertropia) due to recently acquired weakness of a single vertically acting muscle, then determine the weak muscle by performing the Parks-Bielschowsky three-step test (Figure 6-4)

1. The medial and lateral rectus muscles do not have vertical action

2. Therefore, hypertropia (HT) of paretic etiology is caused by weakness of one or more of the following eight vertically acting muscles:

   a. Right inferior oblique (RIO); left inferior oblique (LIO)

   b. Right superior oblique (RSO); left superior oblique (LSO)

   c. Right inferior rectus (RIR); left inferior rectus (LIR)

   d. Right superior rectus (RSR); left superior rectus (LSR)

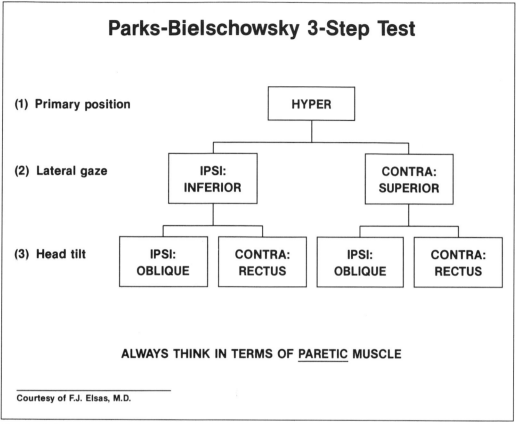

Parks-Bielschowsky 3-Step Test

(1) **Primary position**		**HYPER**

| (2) **Lateral gaze** | **IPSI: INFERIOR** | **CONTRA: SUPERIOR** |

| (3) **Head tilt** | **IPSI: OBLIQUE** | **CONTRA: RECTUS** | **IPSI: OBLIQUE** | **CONTRA: RECTUS** |

ALWAYS THINK IN TERMS OF <u>PARETIC</u> MUSCLE

Courtesy of F.J. Elsas, M.D.

Figure 6-4.

3. If the HT is due to weakness of only one of these eight muscles, the paretic muscle is identified by answering the three questions asked in the Parks-Bielschowsky three-step test
4. Each step cuts the possible number of muscles in half
    a. After the first step, there are four possible muscles remaining
    b. After the second step, there are two remaining
    c. After the third step, only the one guilty muscle remains
5. Parks-Bielschowsky first step: which is the higher eye?
    a. If the patient has a RHT, then the weak muscle is either a depressor of the right eye (RIR, RSO) or an elevator of the left eye (LSR, LIO)
    b. If the patient has a LHT, then the weak muscle is either an elevator of the right eye (RSR, RIO) or a depressor of the left eye (LIR, LSO)
    c. Therefore, by determining if the patient has a RHT or a LHT, you have narrowed down the number of suspected muscles from eight to four
6. Parks-Bielschowsky second step: HT worse on gaze right or left?
    a. The vertical rectus muscles (superior and inferior recti) have their greatest vertical action (and least torsional action) when the eye is abducted

b. Therefore, LHT due to paresis of LIR will be worse on gaze left (since OS is abducted on gaze left); LHT due to paresis of RSR will be worse on gaze right (since OD is abducted on right gaze)

c. The oblique muscles (superior and inferior obliques) have their greatest vertical action (and least torsional action) when the eye is adducted

d. Therefore, LHT due to paresis of LSO will be worse on gaze right; LHT due to paresis of RIO will be worse on gaze left

e. LHT worse on gaze right is due to weakness of either LSO or RSR

f. LHT worse on gaze left is due to weakness of either LIR or RIO

g. Thus, in the case of LHT, by answering the question: "Is LHT worse on gaze right or left?" you have narrowed the possible muscles from four (LSO, RSR, LIR, RIO) to two (either LSO-RSR or LIR-RIO)

h. Similarly, the possible causes of RHT are narrowed down from four (RIR, LIO, LSR, RSO) to two (RIR-LIO if RHT worse on gaze right; LSR-RSO if RHT worse on gaze left). Note: in each case
   i. RHT worse on gaze right (RIR or LIO)
   ii. RHT worse on gaze left (RSO or LSR)
   iii. LHT worse on gaze right (LSO or RSR)
   iv. LHT worse on gaze left (RIO or LIR)
      You are left with either two superior or two inferior muscles; and one will be a rectus and one an oblique, and one will be of the right eye and one of the left. If this is not the case (eg, if you have narrowed it down after the second step to "RIR vs. LSR" or "LSO vs. LIO"), then you have made a mistake and need to retrace your steps

7. Parks-Bielschowsky third step: is the HT worse on head-tilt right (head tilted so that the right ear is near the right shoulder) or head-tilt left (head tilted so that the left ear is near the left shoulder)?

a. The superior muscles (SR and SO) intort the eyes; the inferior muscles (IR and IO) extort the eye

b. When the head is tilted downward to the right shoulder, the eyes undergo corrective torsion (ie, OD intorted and OS extorted)

c. Therefore, when the head is tilted to the right, OD will be intorted by contraction of RSR and RSO; these two muscles work together in affecting the intorsion and neutralize each other's vertical action (RSR is an elevator and RSO a depressor)

d. If one of these muscles is the paretic muscle responsible for the HT, then the vertical action will not be neutralized and the HT will be worse on tilting the head to the right shoulder

e. Therefore, the mnemonic for the third step is:
   i. If you are left with two superior muscles, then the paretic muscle is the one on the same side as the shoulder toward which the head-tilt makes the HT worse (eg, if it is narrowed down to "RSO vs. LSR," then the paretic muscle is "RSO if RHT worse on tilt to right" and "LSR if RHT is worse to tilt left")
   ii. If you are left with two inferior muscles, then the paretic muscle is the one on the side opposite the shoulder toward which the head-tilt makes

the HT worse (eg, if it is narrowed down to "RIO vs. LIR," then the paretic muscle is "RIO if LHT worse on tilt left" and "LIR if LHT worse on tilt right")

B. Bajandas described Bielschowsky's "missing step": Is the HT worse on gaze up or gaze down?

    1. This step confirms step three

    2. Note again that after step two we are down to either two superior or two inferior muscles

        a. RSR vs. LSO

        b. RSO vs. LSR

        c. RIR vs. LIO

        d. RIO vs. LIR

    3. Note also that in each case, one muscle is an elevator and the other a depressor

    4. Therefore, we can confirm the paretic muscle identified by step three by noting if the HT is worse on gaze up (RSR, LSR, LIO, RIO) or gaze down (LSO, RSO, RIR, LIR)

IV. Measuring the torsional component of IV nerve palsy

A. Double Maddox rod test to quantitate torsional component of diplopia

B. The patient will report intorsion of image seen by eye with IV nerve palsy. Actually, this indicates extorsion of the patient's eye caused by overaction of the antagonist inferior oblique muscle (Figure 6-5)

C. Greater than 10 degrees of torsion is suggestive of bilateral IV nerve palsies

V. Bilateral IV nerve palsies

A. Usually due to severe head trauma with contusion of the anterior medullary velum where the IV nerve fascicles cross

B. Parks-Bielschowsky three-step test

    1. Either eye may be hypertropic in primary position or patient may be orthophoric

    2. RHT on gaze left; LHT on gaze right

    3. RHT on head-tilt right; LHT on head-tilt left

C. With double Maddox rods, measure greater than 10 degrees of torsion

VI. Incidence of various causes of IV nerve palsy

A. Table 6-1 summarizes eight large series of patients with acquired paresis of the IV nerve

B. Summary of cases of acquired, isolated IV paresis (10-20-30-40 rule)

    1. 10%: neoplasm-aneurysm

    2. 20%: ischemic

    3. 30%: undetermined or miscellaneous

    4. 40%: trauma

C. A large proportion of IV nerve palsies are classified as congenital. In Harley's series of 18 children, 67% (12/18) were congenital; while in Younge's report of 52 adults, 29% (15/52) were congenital

D. The frequency of congenital IV nerve paresis cannot be overemphasized. Many adults presenting in the fifth and sixth decades of life may have decompensated, congenital IV nerve palsies

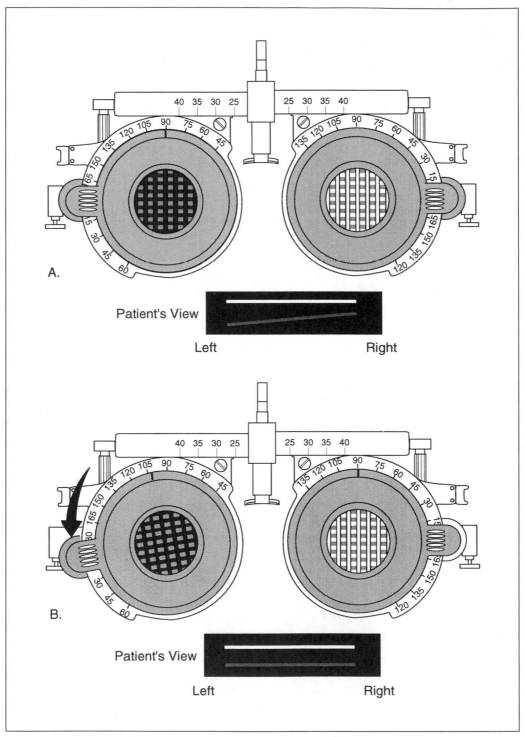

Figure 6-5. Double Maddox rod test for cyclodeviation in a patient with a right IV nerve palsy. A red and white Maddox rod is inserted into a trial frame, with the red lens before the eye with a suspected cyclodeviation. Special care must be taken to align the direction of the glass rods with the 90-degree mark of the trial frame. The trial frame must be adjusted carefully to a more exact horizontal position (modified from Van Noorden GK. *Atlas of Strabismus.* 4th ed. St. Louis, Mo: CV Mosby; 1983: 52-53).

Table 6-1

ETIOLOGIES OF ACQUIRED IV NERVE PALSY

	Rucker (1958)	Rucker (1966)	Khawam (1967)	Burger (1970)	Younge (1977)	Rush (1981)	Kodsi (1992) (children)	Richards (1992)
Total # Patients	67	84	40	33	36	172	19	248
Etiologies (%)								
Neoplasm	4	8	2.5	21	0	4	5	4
Trauma	36	27	67.5	39	44	32	37	26
Aneurysm	0	0	0	3	0	2	0	1
Ischemic	36	15	2.5	18	33	18	0	14
Miscellaneous	10	15	7.5	9	8	4	37	20
Undetermined	13	33	20	6	15	36	21	35

VII. Differential diagnosis of vertical diplopia

    A. Ocular myasthenia

    B. Thyroid eye disease

    C. Orbital disease (tumor, trauma, inflammation, blowout fracture of the floor)

    D. III nerve paresis

    E. Brown's syndrome

    F. Skew deviation

VIII. Other syndromes of the superior oblique muscle

    A. Brown's (sheath) syndrome

        1. Limitation of elevation of the eye in adduction because movements of the superior oblique tendon in the trochlea are restricted

        2. Affected eyes usually hypotropic, and the patient often develops abnormal head position (chin up)

        3. Forced ductions must be positive to establish diagnosis

        4. Congenital etiology: superior oblique tendon is short and tethered

        5. Acquired etiologies:

            a. Tenosynovitis may prevent tendon from passing through the trochlear pulley

            b. Orbital trauma to trochlear region

    B. Superior oblique myokymia

        1. Unexplained condition causing vertical diplopia or monocular blurred vision with tremulous sensations of the affected eye

        2. Paroxysmal, rapid, vertical, and torsional movements of one eye that are usually small, necessitating slit lamp examination or ophthalmoscopy

        3. Precipitated by asking the patient to first look in the direction of action of the superior oblique muscle and then return to the primary position

        4. Usually benign; occasionally seen with multiple sclerosis or posterior fossa tumor

        5. Treatment:

            a. Carbamazepine (Tegretol); propranolol (Inderal)

            b. Superior oblique surgery

Bibliography

Chapters

Glaser JS, Siatkowski RM. Infranuclear disorders of eye movements. In: Duane TD, ed. *Duane's Clinical Ophthalmology*. Vol 2. Philadelphia, Pa: Lippincott-Williams & Wilkins; 1998: chapter 12, 1-63.

Leigh RJ, Zee DS. *The Neurology of Eye Movements*. 3rd ed. New York, NY: Oxford University Press; 1999: 321-404.

Smith C. Nuclear and infranuclear ocular motility disorders. In: Miller NR, Newman NJ, eds. *Walsh and Hoyt's Clinical Neuro-ophthalmology*. Vol 1. 5th ed. Baltimore, Md: Williams & Wilkins; 1998: 1189-1281.

Articles

Brazis PW. Palsies of the trochlear nerve: diagnosis and localization—recent concepts. *Mayo Clin Proc.* 1993;68:501-509.

Brown HW. True and simulated superior oblique tendon sheath syndromes. *Doc Ophthalmol.* 1973;34:123-136.

Burger LJ, Kalvin NH, Smith JL. Acquired lesions of the fourth cranial nerve. *Brain.* 1970;93:567-574.

Coppeto IR. Superior oblique paresis and contralateral Horner's syndrome. *Ann Ophthalmol.* 1983;681-683.

Harley RD. Paralytic strabismus in children: etiologic incidence and management of the third, fourth, and sixth nerve palsies. *Ophthalmology.* 1980;86:24-43.

Hoyt WF, Keane JR. Superior oblique myokymia: report and discussion on five cases of benign intermittent uniocular microtremor. *Arch Ophthalmol.* 1970;84:461-467.

Jacobson DM, Warner JJ, Choucair AK, Ptacek LJ. Trochlear nerve palsy following minor head trauma. A sign of structural disorder. *J Clin Neuro-ophthalmol.* 1988;8:263-268.

Kodsi SR, Younge BR. Acquired oculomotor trochlear and abducent cranial nerve palsies in pediatric patients. *Am J Ophthalmol.* 1992;114:568-574.

Morrow MJ, Sharpe JA, Ranalli PJ. Superior oblique myokymia associated with a posterior fossa tumor: oculographic correlation with an idiopathic case. *Neurology.* 1990;40:367-370.

Moster ML, Bosley TM, Slavin ML, Rubin SE. Thyroid ophthalmopathy presenting as superior oblique palsies. *J Clin Neuro-ophthalmol.* 1992;12:94-97.

Parks MM. Isolated cyclovertical muscle palsy. *Arch Ophthalmol.* 1958;60:1027-1035.

Richards BW, Jones FR, Younge BR. Cause and prognoses of 4278 cases of paralysis of oculomotor, trochlear and abducens cranial nerves. *Am J Ophthalmol.* 1992;183:489-496.

Rucker CW. Paralysis of the third, fourth, and sixth cranial nerves. *Am J Ophthalmol.* 1958;46:787-794.

Rucker CW. The causes of paralysis of the third, fourth, and sixth cranial nerves. *Am J Ophthalmol.* 1966;61:1293-1298.

Rush JA, Younge BR. Paralysis of cranial nerves III, IV, and VI. Cause and prognosis in 1,000 cases. *Arch Ophthalmol.* 1981;99:76-79.

Spector RH. Vertical diplopia. *Surv Ophthalmol.* 1993;38:31-62.

Susac JO, Smith JL, Schatz NJ. Superior oblique myokymia. *Arch Neurol.* 1973;29:432-434.

Younge BR, Sutula F. Analysis of trochlear nerve palsies: diagnosis, etiology, and treatment. *Mayo Clinic Proc.* 1977;52:11-18.

Chapter 7

Cavernous Sinus Syndrome

I. **General considerations**

　A. The ocular motor cranial nerves lie in proximity within the cavernous sinus and superior orbital fissure

　B. Since the cavernous sinus contains structures that continue through the superior orbital fissure, it is often impossible to state whether a lesion is in the sinus or in the fissure. More general designation is parasellar syndrome

　C. Typically, patients present with periorbital or hemicranial pain, combined with ipsilateral ocular motor cranial nerve palsies, oculosympathetic paralysis, and sensory loss in the distribution of the ophthalmic (V^1) and occasionally maxillary (V^2) division of the trigeminal nerve. Clinically, various combinations of these cranial nerve palsies occur

　D. The "orbital apex syndrome" should be reserved for multiple ocular motor cranial nerve palsies plus optic nerve dysfunction

II. **Anatomy (Figures 7-1 and 7-2)**

　A. Traditionally, the cavernous sinus was thought to be an unbroken, trabeculated structure, but recent studies demonstrate that it is a plexus of various-sized veins that divide and coalesce

　B. Major constituents:

　　　1. III nerve
　　　2. IV nerve
　　　3. VI nerve
　　　4. Ophthalmic nerve (V^1)
　　　5. Sympathetic carotid plexus
　　　6. Intracavernous carotid artery

　C. The III, IV, V^1 nerves all lie in a lateral wall of the cavernous sinus. The VI nerve lies freely within the sinus, just lateral to the intracavernous carotid

III. **Causes of cavernous sinus syndrome producing painful ophthalmoplegia**

　A. Trauma

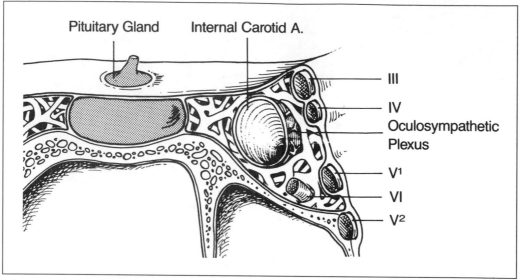

Figure 7-1. Coronal view of the left cavernous sinus and its contents.

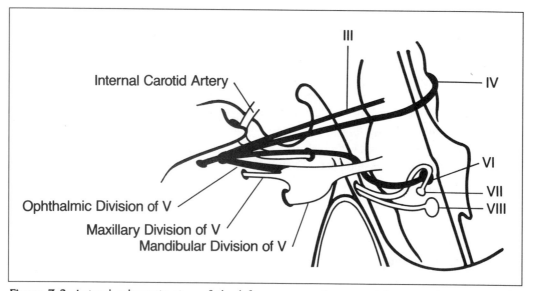

Figure 7-2. Lateral schematic view of the left cavernous sinus; cranial nerves that traverse the sinus are highlighted in black.

    B. Vascular

        1. Intracavernous carotid artery aneurysm

        2. Posterior cerebral artery aneurysm

        3. Carotid-cavernous fistula

        4. Carotid-cavernous thrombosis

    C. Neoplasm

1. Primary intracranial tumor
   a. Pituitary adenoma
   b. Meningioma
   c. Craniopharyngioma
   d. Sarcoma
   e. Neurofibroma
   f. Gasserian ganglion neuroma
   g. Epidermoid
   h. Hemangioma/hemangiopericytoma
   i. Eosinophilic granuloma
2. Primary cranial tumor
   a. Chordoma
   b. Chondroma
   c. Giant-cell tumor
3. Local metastases
   a. Nasopharyngeal tumor
   b. Cylindroma
   c. Adamantinoma
   d. Squamous cell carcinoma
4. Distant metastases
   a. Lymphoma
   b. Multiple myeloma
   c. Carcinomatous metastases

D. Inflammation
   1. Bacterial: sinusitis, mucocele, periostitis
   2. Viral: herpes zoster
   3. Fungal: mucormycosis
   4. Spirochetal: treponema pallidum
   5. Mycobacterial: mycobacterium tuberculosis
   6. Unknown cause: sarcoidosis, Wegener's granulomatosis, Tolosa-Hunt syndrome

IV. **Of the more common causes of cavernous sinus syndrome, these points deserve emphasis:**

A. Intracavernous carotid artery aneurysm
   1. Typically produces slowly progressive, unilateral ophthalmoplegia
   2. May become painful
   3. Rarely rupture, but this occurrence produces a carotid-cavernous fistula

B. Carotid-cavernous fistula
   1. Due to direct communication between intracavernous carotid artery and cavernous sinus
   2. High-flow, high-pressure fistula
   3. Most common cause is head trauma
   4. Clinical picture: chemosis, proptosis, ocular motor nerve palsies, bruit, retinopathy, increased intraocular pressure

C. Dural-cavernous fistula
1. Due to communication of dural branches of internal or external carotid arteries and cavernous sinus or vessels in region of sinus
2. Low-flow, low-pressure fistula
3. Most commonly occur spontaneously
4. More subtle clinical picture: don't be fooled into treating these patients for "red eye"
5. On occasion, fistula flow is directed posteriorly, causing chronic ocular motor cranial nerve palsies without orbital congestive signs ("white-eyed shunt")

D. Nasopharyngeal carcinoma
1. Two to three times more common in males
2. Predilection for Asian patients
3. Varied clinical presentation
   a. Nasal obstruction
   b. Rhinorrhea
   c. Epistaxis
   d. Otitis media
   e. Proptosis
   f. Ipsilateral dry eye
4. Ninety-five percent of patients with nasopharyngeal carcinoma have VI nerve paresis at some time during clinical course
5. Radiologic study of choice: cranial magnetic resonance (MR) scanning with attention to subcranial soft tissue in region of nasopharynx
6. Indirect pharyngoscopy and biopsies of the nasopharynx if clinical suspicion high

E. Two aspects of neoplastic involvement of the parasellar region require particular attention
1. Mode of onset and clinical course do not prognosticate the type of lesion (ie, neoplastic disease may have an acute clinical presentation as well as an expected insidious course)
2. High-dose corticosteroid therapy may initially improve signs and symptoms due to neoplasm

F. Tolosa-Hunt syndrome
1. Painful ophthalmoplegia due to granulomatous inflammation occurring in the cavernous sinus
2. Spontaneous remissions may occur after days or weeks
3. Recurring attacks may occur at intervals of months or years
4. Systemic steroids usually lead to marked improvement of signs and symptoms within 48 hours
5. Categorically, diagnosis of exclusion and patients with this diagnosis require careful follow-up

V. **Imitators of cavernous sinus syndrome**

A. Myasthenia
B. Ocular dysthyroidism
C. Orbital disease: inflammation, infection, neoplasm, trauma
D. Diabetic ophthalmoplegia

1. Typically acute, often painful, mononeuropathy with full recovery within 4 months
2. Less frequent occurrence of simultaneous paralysis of multiple ocular motor nerves. Often painful, recurrent, and not responsive to steroid therapy

E. Giant cell arteritis
   1. Single or multiple ocular motor nerve palsies
   2. Produces ischemic necrosis of extraocular muscles

F. Botulism
   1. Occurs in three forms: food-borne, wound, infantile
   2. Ophthalmologic findings include dilated, poorly reactive pupils, ptosis, and ophthalmoplegia
   3. Affected individuals have nausea, vomiting, associated with facial, pharyngeal, and generalized proximal weakness, and no sensory deficits
   4. Botulinum toxin is the most potent poison known, causing cholinergic blockade with only minute quantities

G. Fisher's syndrome
   1. Bulbar variant of Guillain-Barré syndrome, characterized by triad of ataxia, areflexia, ophthalmoplegia
   2. In evolution, this cranial polyneuropathy may mimic unilateral or bilateral ocular motor cranial nerve palsies, but usually progresses to a virtually total ophthalmoplegia with involvement of pupils and accommodation
   3. Patients may also have facial diplegia, respiratory and swallowing difficulties, and confusion
   4. Often follows a febrile or "viral" illness
   5. Over 90% of patients have antibodies to the ganglioside GQ1b
   6. Patients frequently have "albumino-cytologic" dissociation on examination of cerebrospinal fluid (ie, elevated protein in the absence of a pleocytosis)

BIBLIOGRAPHY

Chapters

Parkinson D. Anatomy of the cavernous sinus. In: Smith JL, ed. *Neuro-ophthalmology.* Vol 6. St. Louis, Mo: CV Mosby; 1972:73-101.

Schatz NJ, Farmer P. Tolosa-Hunt syndrome: the pathology of painful ophthalmoplegia. In: Smith JL, ed. *Neuro-ophthalmology.* Vol 6. St. Louis, Mo: CV Mosby; 1972:102-112.

Articles

Acieino M, Trobe JD, Cornbluth WT, Gebarski SS. Painful oculomotor palsy caused by posterior-draining dural carotid cavernous fistulas. *Arch Ophthalmol.* 1995;113:1045-1049.

Barricks ME, Traviesa DB, Glaser JS, et al. Ophthalmoplegia in giant cell arteries. *Brain.* 1977;100:209-221.

Chiba A, Kusonoki S, Obata H, Machinumi R, Kanazana I. Serum anti-GQ1b antibody is associated with ophthalmoplegia in Miller Fisher syndrome and Guillain-Barré syndrome: clinical and immunohistochemical studies. *Neurology.* 1993;43:1911-1917.

Fisher CM. An unusual variant of acute idiopathic polyneuritis (syndrome of ophthalmoplegia, ataxia, areflexia). *N Engl J Med.* 1956;255:57-65.

Harris FS, Rhoton AL. Anatomy of the cavernous sinus. A microsurgical study. *J Neurosurg.* 1976;45:169-180.

Hedges TR III, Jones A, Stark L, et al. Botulin ophthalmoplegia: clinical and oculographic observation. *Arch Ophthalmol.* 1983;101:211-213.

Hunt WE, Meagher JN, LeFever HE, et al. Painful ophthalmoplegia: its relation to indolent inflammation of the cavernous sinus. *Neurology.* 1961;11:56-62.

Kline LB. The Tolosa-Hunt syndrome. *Surv Ophthalmol.* 1982;27:79-95.

Meadows SP. Intracavernous aneurysm of the internal carotid artery in the cavernous sinus. *Arch Ophthalmol.* 1959;62:566-574.

Newton TH, Hoyt WF. Dural arteriovenous shunts in the region of the cavernous sinus. *Neuroradiology.* 1970;1:71-81.

Sanders MD, Hoyt WF. Hypoxic ocular sequelae of carotid-cavernous fistulae. *Br J Ophthalmol.* 1969;53:82-97.

Sergott RC, Grossman RI, Savino PJ, Bosley TM, Schatz NJ. The syndrome of paradoxical worsening of dural-cavernous sinus arteriovenous malformations. *Ophthalmology.* 1987;94:205-221.

Smith JL, Taxdal DSR. Painful ophthalmoplegia: the Tolosa-Hunt syndrome. *Am J Ophthalmol.* 1966;61:1466-1472.

Thomas JE, Yoss RE. The parasellar syndrome: problems in determining etiology. *Mayo Clin Proc.* 1970;45:617-623.

Tolosa E. Periarteritic lesions of the carotid siphon with the clinical features of a carotid infraclinoid aneurysm. *J Neurol Neurosurg Psychiatry.* 1954;17:300-302.

Trobe JD, Glaser JS, Post MJD. Meningiomas and aneurysms of the cavernous sinus. *Arch Ophthalmol.* 1978;96:457-467.

Warren FA. Diagnosis and management of cavernous sinus lesions. *Ophthalmol Clin NA.* 1991;4:605-613.

Chapter 8

The Pupil

I.   Anatomical considerations

   A. Sphincter muscle of the iris

     1. Innervated by parasympathetic fibers originating in the Edinger-Westphal (EW) nucleus, which forms part of the oculomotor nuclear complex in the midbrain

     2. Input that excites the EW nucleus

       a. Light reflex (Figure 8-1)

         i. Afferent neurons from retinal ganglion cells to the pretectal area; intercalated neurons from the pretectal complex to EW nuclei; parasympathetic outflow with the oculomotor nerve to the ciliary ganglion and then to the iris sphincter muscle

         ii. Monocular light information is carried by the optic nerve to the chiasm, where approximately half the fibers decussate to the contralateral optic tract, and half the fibers continue in the ipsilateral optic tract

         iii. Approximately two-thirds of the way along the optic tract, some of the axons leave the tract, enter the brachium of the superior colliculus, and synapse in the pretectal region

         iv. The information is then passed forward via the intercalated neurons to the EW nuclei bilaterally

         v. The pupillomotor information travels with the III nerve and through the superior orbital fissure with the inferior division

         iv. Thus, light information received by one eye is transmitted to both pupils equally

       b. Near synkinesis (Figure 8-2)

         i. The peristriate cortex (area 19), at the upper end of the calcarine fissure, may be the origin of near synkinesis

         ii. Near synkinesis triad

           a. Convergence of eyes

           b. Accommodation of the lenses

           c. Miosis of the pupils

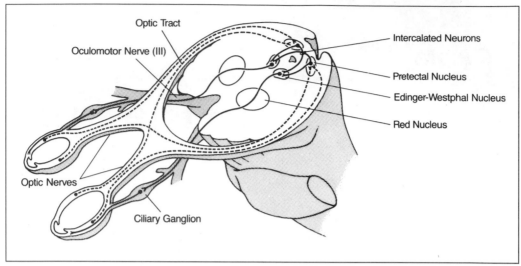

Figure 8-1. Pathway of the pupillary light reflex (redrawn from Miller NR. *Walsh and Hoyt's Clinical Neuro-ophthalmology.* 4th ed. Vol 2. Baltimore, Md: Williams & Wilkins; 1985: 421).

        iii. The near synkinesis pathway is more ventrally located than the pretectal afferent limb of the light reflex. This separation of the "near" from "light" reflexes may be the anatomical basis for some instances of light-near dissociation of the pupils (eg, Argyll Robertson pupils, dorsal midbrain syndrome)

        iv. The final pathway is the oculomotor nerve, ciliary ganglion, and the short posterior ciliary nerves. The ratio of ciliary ganglion cells that innervate the ciliary muscle versus cells related to iris sphincter is approximately 30:1

    3. Input that inhibits EW nucleus

        a. Cortical: dilated pupils during epileptic seizures

        b. Spinal-reticular: states of arousal, excitement

        c. Sleep, coma: inhibitory influences decline and pupils are miotic

  B. Dilator muscle of the iris

    1. Innervated by sympathetic fibers

    2. Three neuron pathways (Figure 8-3):

        a. First-order neuron originates in posterior hypothalamus and courses down through the brainstem to the C8-T2 level of the cord (ciliospinal center of Budge)

        b. Second-order (preganglionic) neurons leave the cord, enter the paravertebral sympathetic chain, and terminate in the superior cervical ganglion at the base of the skull

        c. Third-order (postganglionic) neuron fibers intended for the pupil and Muller's muscle ascend the internal carotid artery to enter the skull, join the ophthalmic nerve in the cavernous sinus, and then to the orbit through the superior orbital fissure; the sudomotor and vasomotor fibers to the face travel with the external carotid artery

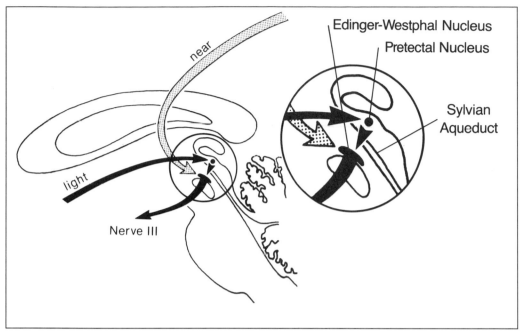

Figure 8-2. Illustration of a more ventral course of near response input (hatched arrow) to EW nucleus compared to light response input (solid arrow).

II. Normal pupillary phenomena

A. Physiologic anisocoria

    1. Approximately 20% of the general population have clearly perceptible (generally less than 0.5 mm) anisocoria. The degree of anisocoria can vary from day to day and even switch sides

B. Pupillary unrest

    1. During distance fixation and with constant, moderate, ambient illumination, the pupils will be noted to have bilaterally, symmetrically, nonrhythmical unrest or variation in size, usually less than 1 mm in amplitude of variation. This is termed hippus

C. Near synkinesis

    1. With sufficient ambient illumination to allow visualization in the pupils, the patient is asked to shift fixation from the distant object to a near point, preferably the patient's own forefinger. Equal miosis of both pupils will be noted

    2. After shifting fixation back to the distant object and maintaining the same ambient illumination, a bright light is placed before one or both eyes and the miosis of the light reflex is noted and compared to the "near" miosis. The "light" miosis will be equal to or greater than the "near" miosis

    3. If a patient demonstrates normal reactions of the pupil to light, there is usually no clinical observation to be gained by testing the near response

D. Psychosensory reflex

    1. While maintaining constant "near" and "light" stimuli, the examiner observes pupillary size with the use of a "startle" stimulus, such as a loud noise or pain

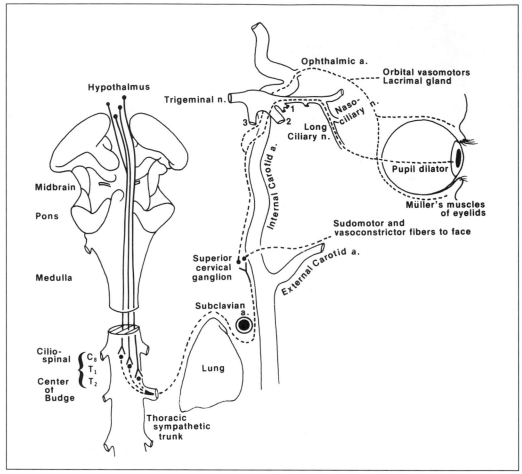

Figure 8-3. Diagram of oculosympathetic pathway (reprinted with permission from Glaser JS. The pupils and accommodation. In: Duane TD, ed. *Clinical Ophthalmology.* Vol 2. Philadelphia, Pa: Lippincott-Williams & Wilkins; 1994: chapter 15, 5).

    2. The pupils will dilate due to two neural mechanisms
        a. Active sympathetic discharges (stimulate iris dilator muscle)
        b. Inhibition of ocular motor nuclei (relaxation of iris sphincter muscle)
    3. The psychosensory reflex is helpful when demonstrating Horner's syndrome

E. Direct pupillary light reflex
    1. By having the subject fixate on a distant object (thereby obviating the miosis associated with accommodation) and the ambient illumination moderately subdued, the direct pupillary response is noted when a bright light is placed before one eye
    2. The pupil constricts briskly, with a subsequent slow dilation to an intermediate size, followed by a state of pupillary unrest (hippus)
    3. The normalcy of the briskness and the latency of the initial response can be evaluated by clinical experience but will be further evaluated by comparison with the fellow eye during the direct light reflex test as well as during the swinging flashlight test (see next page)

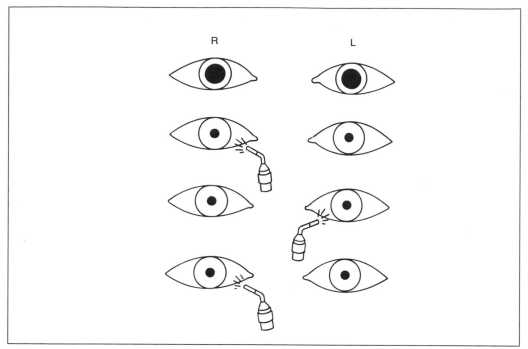

Figure 8-4. Normal response to swinging flashlight test with no change in size of pupils.

4. The amplitudes of the initial constriction and subsequent redilation (pupillary escape) depend upon the ambient illumination and the relative brightness of the test light. These amplitudes are also subject to marked individual variation and are best evaluated by comparison with the fellow eye during the swinging flashlight test

F. Consensual pupillary reflex

1. Because of the equal distribution (to both III nerves) of the photic information provided by one eye, the fellow pupil will behave in the same manner described above for the direct light reflex

G. Swinging flashlight test (Figure 8-4)

1. While maintaining the same test conditions described in testing the direct pupillary light reflex, the examiner projects the light on (for example) the right eye and allows the right to go through the phase of initial constriction to a minimum size and subsequent escape to an intermediate size

2. At this point, the examiner quickly swings the light to the left eye, which will begin at the intermediate size and go through the phases of initial constriction to a minimum size and subsequent escape to an intermediate size

3. As soon as the left pupil redilates to the intermediate size, the light is swung to the right eye and a mental note made of the intermediate (starting) size, the latency and briskness of the response, the minimum size, the latency and briskness of the redilation of the intermediate size

4. These characteristics will be exactly the same in both eyes as the light is alternately swung to each eye

5. Key points in proper testing:

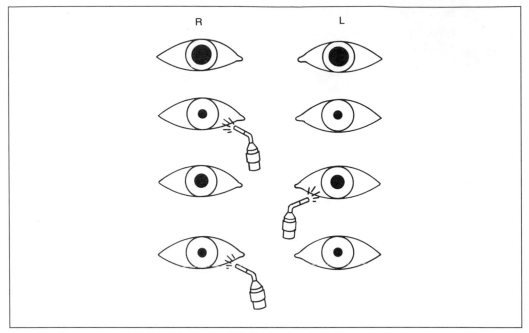

Figure 8-5. Afferent pupillary defect in the left eye using a swinging flashlight test. The pupils constrict when the light is shined in the right eye; however, when the flashlight is swung back to the left eye, both pupils dilate.

   a. A bright hand light in a darkened room is essential
   b. The patient should fix on a distant object
   c. The light should cross from one eye to the other fairly rapidly (across the bridge of the nose) and remain 3 to 5 seconds on each eye to allow pupillary stabilization

III. Abnormal pupillary states

   A. Afferent pupillary defect (Marcus Gunn pupil) (Figure 8-5)
      1. During the swinging flashlight test, if the amount of light information transmitted from one eye is less than that carried from the fellow eye, the following phenomenon may be noted when the light is swung from the normal eye to the defective eye
         a. Immediate dilation of the pupil, instead of normal initial constriction (3 to 4+ Marcus Gunn pupil)
         b. No change in pupil size initially, followed by dilation of the pupils (1 to 2+ Marcus Gunn pupil)
         c. Initial constriction, but greater escape to a larger intermediate size than when the light is swung back to the normal eye (trace Marcus Gunn pupil)
      2. When the light is swung back to the normal eye, the pupil demonstrates the normal pattern of brisk constriction (of short latency) with subsequent escape to an intermediate size
      3. Optic neuropathy (must be unilateral or markedly asymmetric) will usually present with a significant Marcus Gunn pupil
      4. Opacities of the ocular media (corneal scar, cataract, vitreous hemorrhage) will not cause a Marcus Gunn pupillary phenomenon if a strong enough flashlight is used

5. Maculopathy, or amblyopic "lazy eye," will not cause a Marcus Gunn phenomenon unless very extensive (less than 20/200 acuity) and then it will only be a 1+ phenomenon, compared to a 3 to 4+ if the 20/200 acuity was due to an optic neuropathy

6. Extensive retinal damage will cause a significant Marcus Gunn phenomenon

7. Amaurotic pupil: the maximum Marcus Gunn pupil imaginable; seen in patients with "blind eye"

8. There is no such thing as "bilateral" Marcus Gunn pupils; there may be bilaterally reduced direct response of the pupils to light, resulting in "light-near" dissociation, but the Marcus Gunn phenomenon requires asymmetry of the afferent light transmission

9. Isolated, unilateral optic neuropathy does not cause the ipsilateral pupil to be larger; the pupils remain the same size because of the consensual reflex. Unilateral amaurotic mydriasis does not exist

10. Detection of the afferent pupillary defect requires only one "working" pupil. If one pupil is mechanically or pharmacologically nonreactive, one can simply perform a swinging flashlight test observing the reactive pupil. If the abnormal eye is the eye with a fixed pupil, then the pupil of the normal eye will constrict briskly when the light is shined directly in it and will dilate when the light is shined in the opposite eye. If the abnormal eye is the eye with the reactive pupil, then the pupil will constrict when light is shined in the opposite eye and will dilate when the light is shined directly in it

B. Adie's tonic pupil

1. Idiopathic, benign cause of internal ophthalmoplegia

2. Eighty percent unilateral initially; tends to become bilateral at a rate of 4% per year

3. Female predilection (70% vs. 30%)

4. Young adults: 20 to 40 years of age

5. Dilated pupil with poor to absent light reaction

6. Slow constriction to prolonged near-effort and slow redilation (tonic response) after near effort

7. Most patients initially have accommodative paresis, which usually resolves over several months

8. Primary finding of segmental palsy of iris sphincter muscle

9. Adie's pupil frequently (80% of cases) demonstrates cholinergic supersensitivity to weak pilocarpine solutions (0.125% or 0.10%)

10. Etiology in most cases is unknown. Lesion causing Adie's pupil located in the ciliary ganglion or short posterior ciliary nerves; aberrant regeneration of more numerous fibers innervating the ciliary muscle (97%) into those subserving the iris sphincter muscle (3%)

11. Adie's syndrome: pupillary abnormalities occurring in a patient with associated diminished deep tendon reflexes

C. Argyll Robertson pupils

1. Miotic, irregular pupils

2. Absence of pupillary light response associated with normal anterior visual pathway function

3. Brisk pupillary constriction to near stimuli

4. Poor dilation in the dark and in response to mydriatic agents

5. Condition is usually bilateral, but is often asymmetric and may be unilateral

6. Etiology: major consideration is neurosyphilis. Other reported causes include diabetes mellitus, chronic alcoholism, multiple sclerosis, sarcoidosis

7. Site of lesion: most likely in the region of the Sylvian aqueduct in the rostral midbrain interfering with the light reflex fibers and supranuclear inhibitory fibers as they approach the EW nuclei. More ventrally located fibers for near response are spared (see Figure 8-2)

D. Light-near dissociation of the pupils

    1. Better pupillary response to "near" than to "light"

    2. Differential diagnosis

        a. Optic neuropathy or severe retinopathy (probably most common cause)

        b. Adie's tonic pupil

        c. Argyll Robertson pupils

        d. Dorsal midbrain syndrome

        e. Aberrant regeneration of III nerve; defective response to light with aberrent hook-up of medial rectus fibers to the pupillary fibers, resulting in pupillary constriction during adduction

        f. Miscellaneous causes: amyloidosis, diabetes, Dejerine-Sottas, Charcot-Marie-Tooth

E. The pupils of coma

    1. Hutchinson pupil

        a. Comatose patient with unilaterally dilated, poorly reactive pupil

        b. Probably due to ipsilateral, expanding, intracranial, supratentorial mass (eg, tumor, subdural hematoma) that is causing downward displacement of hippocampal gyrus and uncal herniation across the tentorial edge with entrapment of the III nerve (see Figure 5-4)

        c. The pupillomotor fibers travel in the peripheral portion of the III nerve (near the perineurium) and are subject to early damage from compression

    2. Miosis

        a. During the early stages of coma, the cortical inhibitory input to the EW nucleus is diminished and the pupils are small but reactive to light

        b. Remember pharmacologic miosis

            i. Morphine

            ii. Pilocarpine: if the patient is being incidentally treated for glaucoma

F. The pupils of hospital personnel (pharmacologic blockade)

    1. Unilaterally dilated, fixed pupil

    2. Due to inadvertent contact with mydriatic agent, most commonly atropine

G. Traumatic pupil

    1. Contusion injury of the eye may cause miosis or mydriasis

    2. Miosis may be due to sphincter spasm seen with iritis

    3. Mydriasis may be due to contusion injury (or actual rupture) of the iris sphincter muscle

        a. Irregular pupil

        b. Poorly responsive to 1% pilocarpine

H. Pharmacologic differentiation of the causes of a fixed, dilated pupil
 1. The patient is tested first with 0.1% pilocarpine, then, if necessary, 1% pilocarpine
 2. If the pupil constricts to 0.1% pilocarpine, then the patient has Adie's pupil; if there is no response to 0.1% pilocarpine, then proceed to 1%
 3. If 1% pilocarpine constricts the involved pupil, then the patient may have a III nerve paresis
 4. If 1% pilocarpine fails to constrict the involved pupil, or does so poorly, the patient has either pharmacologic blockade or a traumatic pupil

I. Horner's syndrome (oculosympathetic paralysis)
 1. Three neuron pathways (see Figure 8-3)
 2. Clinical signs:
     a. Miosis of the affected pupil, which is more marked in dim illumination (evoking dilation) than in bright illumination
     b. Ptosis of the upper lid; usually 2 to 3 mm
     c. Upside-down ptosis of the low lid (due to paresis of inferior tarsal muscle), causing the lower lid to rest 1 to 2 mm higher on the affected side
     d. Apparent enophthalmos due to narrow palpebral fissure
     e. Anhydrosis of the affected side of the face. This occurs only if the lesion involves the sympathetic pathway proximal to the bifurcation of the common carotid artery, since the sudomotor fibers travel with the external carotid artery
     f. Heterochromia of the affected iris. Characteristic of congenital Horner's with the affected eye having a lighter color
     g. Transient findings
         i. Dilated conjunctival and facial vessels
         ii. Decreased intraocular pressure
         iii. Increased accommodation
 3. Diagnostic steps in suspected Horner's syndrome
     a. Amount of anisocoria should increase in dim versus bright illumination. If this step seems inconclusive, then proceed to cocaine test
     b. Cocaine test
         i. Cocaine (4% to 10%) eyedrops creating sympathomimetic effect by blocking the receptors of norepinephrine at the myoneural junction, thereby prolonging the action of norepinephrine upon the dilator muscle
         ii. Therefore, cocaine requires release of norepinephrine at the myoneural junction by a normal functioning oculosympathetic pathway
         iii. Cocaine drops result in dilation of the normal pupil
         iv. If there is a lesion involving any of the three neurons, pupillary inequality will increase, and the presence of Horner's syndrome is confirmed
     c. Paredrine test
         i. Paredrine (1% hydroxyamphetamine) eyedrops create a sympathomimetic effect by causing release of norepinephrine from the nerve endings at the myoneural junction, thereby stimulating the dilator muscle
         ii. Paredrine requires that the third-order (postganglionic) neuron be intact and have normal axoplasmic activity, including formation and transfer of norepinephrine to the nerve ending at the myoneural junction

iii. Paredrine drops result in dilation of the normal pupil

iv. If there is a lesion of the third-order neuron, there will be subnormal dilation of the pupil by Paredrine

v. Pupillary dilation to Paredrine drops will be normal if the Horner's syndrome is due to lesions of the first- or second-order neurons

d. Therefore, cocaine serves to confirm the presence of Horner's syndrome and Paredrine serves to identify Horner's due to lesions of the third-order neuron

e. Beware of pseudo-Horner's syndrome: ipsilateral ptosis and miosis of unrelated cause

4. Differentiation of causes of Horner's syndrome

a. First-order neuron lesion (brainstem and spinal cord)

i. Cerebrovascular accident (Wallenberg's syndrome)

ii. Neck trauma

iii. Neoplasm

iv. Demyelinating disease

v. Syringomyelia

b. Second-order neuron lesion (preganglionic)

i. Chest lesions: occult carcinoma of the lung apex (Pancoast's tumor), mediastinal mass, cervical rib

ii. Neck lesions: trauma, abscess, thyroid neoplasm, lymphadenopathy

iii. Surgery: thyroidectomy, radical neck surgery, carotid angiography (direct carotid puncture)

c. Third-order neuron lesion (postganglionic)

i. Lesion may be extracranial (similar etiologies as listed for second-order neuron neck lesions) or cause may be intracranial

ii. Migraine variants: cluster headaches, Raeder's paratrigeminal neuralgia

iii. Complicated otitis media

iv. Cavernous sinus/superior orbital fissure lesion

v. Internal carotid artery dissection

vi. Carotid-cavernous fistula

vii. Nasopharyageal carcinoma

5. Horner's syndrome in children

a. Horner's syndrome present at birth usually benign and associated with heterochromia

b. Usually idiopathic (30% to 70%); may be associated with birth trauma (brachial plexus injury); rarely due to intrauterine neuroblastoma

c. Second-order neuron lesion (eg, chest tumor) often behaves pharmacologically like third-order neuron lesion (fails to dilate to hydroxyamphetamine). Probably due to transsynaptic degeneration of preganglionic neuron

d. Acquired Horner's syndrome in first 5 years of life is a more ominous occurrence; often due to neuroblastoma involving sympathetic chain in chest or neck

e. In both congenital and acquired Horner's syndrome, a pediatric evaluation is warranted

IV. Evaluation of a patient with anisocoria (Figure 8-6)

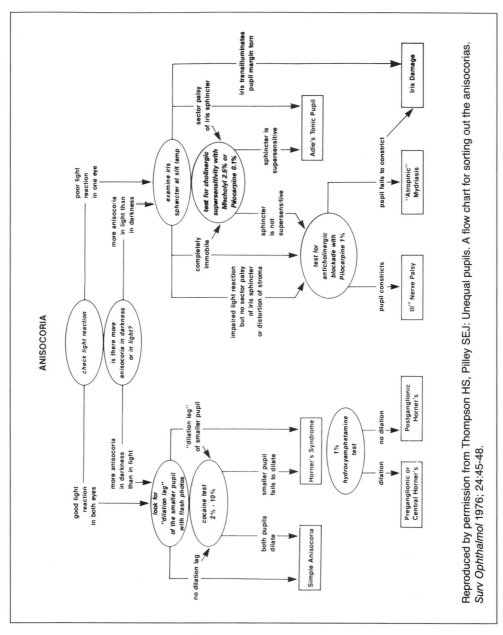

Reproduced by permission from Thompson HS, Pilley SEJ: Unequal pupils. A flow chart for sorting out the anisocorias. *Surv Ophthalmol* 1976; 24:45-48.

Figure 8-6.

V.   Rare pupillary disorders

  A. Benign episodic pupillary dilatation ("springing pupil")
    1. Young, healthy adults
    2. Variable history of migraine
    3. Characteristics:
        a. One pupil widely dilated for minutes to hours
        b. Mild blurring of vision
        c. May have associated periocular discomfort
        d. Headache occurring following episode
    4. Must exclude accidental pharmacologic blockade
    5. Uniformly benign condition

  B. Tadpole pupils
    1. Sectoral pupillary dilation lasting for a few minutes, then returning to normal
    2. Occurs multiple times per day for several days or a week and then disappears
    3. Unusual periocular sensation draws attention to the pupil
    4. Patient may have history of migraine
    5. Possibly due to segmental spasm of iris dilator muscle
    6. Benign condition

  C. Midbrain corectopia
    1. Eccentric or oval pupil seen in patients with rostral midbrain disease
    2. Thought to be due to selective inhibition of iris sphincter tone
    3. Oval pupils may also be seen with midbrain dysfunction due to extrinsic compression from shift of midline supratentorial structures

  D. Paradoxical pupils
    1. Pupillary constriction in darkness
    2. Initially felt to be a sign of retinal disease (congenital stationary night blindness, congenital achromatopsia)
    3. More recently observed in anomalies of optic nerve development (optic nerve coloboma, optic nerve hypoplasia), congenital nystagmus, and a variety of retinal disorders (retinitis pigmentosa, Best's disease, macular dystrophy, albinism)
    4. Mechanism of phenomenon unknown

BIBLIOGRAPHY

Books

Lowenfeld IE. *The Pupil: Anatomy, Physiology and Clinical Applications.* Boston, Mass: Butterworth-Heinemann; 1999.

Chapters

Burde RM, Savino PJ, Trobe JD. *Clinical Decisions in Neuro-ophthalmology.* St. Louis, Mo: Mosby-Year Book; 1992: 321-346.

Glaser JS. Neuro-ophthalmology. In: Duane TD, ed. *Clinical Ophthalmology.* Vol 2. Philadelphia, Pa: Lippincott-Williams & Wilkins; 1998: chapter 15, 1-26.

Kardon RH. Anatomy and physiology of the pupil. In: Miller NR, Newman NJ, eds. *Walsh and Hoyt's Clinical Neuro-ophthalmology.* 5th ed. Vol 1. Baltimore, Md: Williams & Wilkins; 1998: 847-897.

Articles

Cremer SA, Thompson HS, Digre KB, Kardon RH. Hydroxyamphetamine mydriasis in Horner's syndrome. *Am J Ophthalmol.* 1990;110:66-70.

Czarnecki JSC, Thompson HS. The iris sphincter in aberrant regeneration of the third nerve. *Arch Ophthalmol.* 1978;96:1606-1610.

Frank JW, Kushner BJ, France TD. Paradoxic pupillary phenomena. *Arch Ophthalmol.* 1988;106:1564-1566.

Hallett M, Cogan DC. Episodic unilateral mydriasis in otherwise normal patients. *Arch Ophthalmol.* 1970;84:130-136.

Jeffery AR, Ellis FJ, Repka MX, Buncic JR. Pediatric Horner's syndrome. *J Am Ass Ped Ophthalmol Strab.* 1998;2:159-167.

Kardon RH, Denison CE, Brown C, Thompson HS. Critical evaluation of the cocaine test in the diagnosis of Horner's syndrome. *Arch Ophthalmol.* 1990;108:384-387.

Levitan P. Pupillary escape in disease of the retina or optic nerve. *Arch Ophthalmol.* 1959;62:768-779.

Loewenfeld IE. "Simple, central" anisocoria: a common condition, seldom recognized. *Trans Am Acad Ophthalmol Otolaryngol.* 1977;83:832-839.

Loewenfeld IE. The Argyll Robertson pupil, 1869-1969. A critical survey of the literature. *Surv Ophthalmol.* 1969;14:199-299.

Selhorst JB, Hoyt WF, Feinsod M, et al. Midbrain correctopia. *Arch Neurol.* 1976;33:193-195.

Thompson BM, Corbett JJ, Kline LB, et al. Pseudo-Horner's syndrome. *Arch Neurol.* 1982;39:108-111.

Thompson HS. Adie's syndrome: some new observations. *Trans Am Ophthalmol Soc.* 1977;75:587-626.

Thompson HS, Newsome DA, Lowenfeld IE. The fixed dilated pupil: sudden iridoplegia or mydriatic drops? A simple diagnostic test. *Arch Ophthalmol.* 1971;86:21-27.

Thompson HS, Pilley SEJ. Unequal pupils. A flow chart for sorting out the anisocorias. *Surv Ophthalmol.* 1976;21:45-48.

Thompson HS, Zackon DH, Czarnecki JSC. Tadpole-shaped pupils caused by segmental spasm of the iris dilator muscle. *Am J Ophthalmol.* 1983;96:467-472.

Weinstein JM, Zweifel TJ, Thompson HS. Congenital Horner's syndrome. *Arch Ophthalmol.* 1980;98:1074-1078.

Chapter 9

The Swollen Optic Disc

I. **Definitions**

    A. Optic disc edema, swollen disc, "choked" disc: general terms used to describe the optic nerve head affected by a variety of local and systemic causes (Table 9-1)

    B. Papilledema: edema of the optic discs due to increased intracranial pressure being transmitted to the optic nerves by the cerebrospinal fluid (CSF) in the subarachnoid space

II. **Pathophysiology of optic disc edema**

    A. Axonal transport along ganglion cell axons that form the optic nerve occurs in orthograde (cell body to lateral geniculate nucleus) and retrograde (geniculate nucleus to cell body) direction

        1. Orthograde—slow component (1 to 4 mm/day)

        2. Orthograde—fast component (400 mm/day)

        3. Retrograde (200 mm/day)

    B. Accumulation of axoplasmic flow, especially slow orthograde component, at the lamina cribrosa produces disc swelling and nerve fiber layer opacification

    C. In papilledema, increased perineural pressure results in damming of the axoplasmic transport. Other causes of interrupted axonal transport include inflammation (eg, papillitis) and ischemia (eg, ischemic optic neuropathy)

    D. Secondary associated phenomena include dilated retinal veins, exudates, hemorrhages, cotton-wool spots (microinfarcts of the nerve fiber layer)

III. **Papilledema**

    A. Ophthalmoscopic features

        1. Bilateral disc edema (may be asymmetric; rarely unilateral)

        2. Opacification of peripapillary nerve fiber layer

        3. Hyperemia of disc (superficial capillary telangiectasias)

        4. Absent venous pulsations (if venous pulsations are present, then the CSF pressure is probably less than 200 mm of water, 20% of normal patients have absent venous pulsations; therefore, the phenomenon of venous pulsations is helpful only if present)

Table 9-1

CAUSES OF OPTIC DISC EDEMA

Ocular Disease
Uveitis
Hypotony
Vein occlusion

Disc Tumors
Hemangioma
Glioma
Metastatic

Metabolic
Dysthyroidism
Juvenile diabetes
Proliferative retinopathies

Vascular
Ischemic neuropathy
Arteritis, cranial
Arteritis, collagen

Inflammatory
Papillitis
Neuroretinitis
Papillophlebitis
Retrobulbar mass

Orbital Tumors
Perioptic meningioma
Glioma
Sheath "cysts"

Infiltrative
Lymphoma
Reticuloendothelial
Hypertension

Elevated Intracranial Pressure
Mass lesion
Pseudotumor cerebri

Systemic Disease
Anemia
Hypoxemia
Hypertension

Modified from Glaser JS. Neuro-ophthalmology. In: Duane TD, ed. *Clinical Ophthalmology*. Vol 2. Philadelphia, Pa: Lippincott-Williams & Wilkins; 1994: chapter 5, 32.

    5. Splinter hemorrhages (ie, hemorrhages within the nerve fiber layer)

    6. Exudates

    7. Cotton-wool spots

    8. Haziness of the retinal vessels at the disc margins due to swelling of the nerve fiber layer in which the retinal vessels course

    9. Circumferential retinal folds (Paton's lines) in peripapillary region

   10. Obliterated central cup—usually a late finding in papilledema

B. Diagnosis of papilledema constitutes a medical emergency

    1. Cranial computed tomography (CT) or magnetic resonance (MR) scanning to rule out mass lesion

    2. If no mass is discovered and the ventricles are not dilated, CSF analysis to measure opening pressure and look carefully for infectious, infiltrative, or neoplastic cause

C. Visual loss in chronic papilledema

      1. Enlarged blind spots on visual field examination

      2. Transient obscurations of vision, unilateral or bilateral "blacking out" or "graying out" of vision lasting 10 to 15 seconds and recurring many times per day; often precipitated by sudden changes in posture

      3. Gradually, progressive visual field loss, usually beginning nasally and leading to generalized constriction

      4. Chronic atrophic papilledema with eventual loss of central acuity

IV.   Pseudotumor cerebri

A. Four criteria

      1. Increased intracranial pressure

      2. Normal or small-sized ventricles (CT or MR scanning)

      3. Normal CSF composition

      4. Papilledema

B. Patients may complain of headache, transient visual obscurations, diplopia

C. In addition to papilledema, ophthalmologic findings may include.

      1. VI nerve palsy (see VI^2 syndrome in Chapter 4)

      2. Visual field changes (large blind spots, generalized constriction)

D. Patients are frequently young adult, obese females who otherwise report a sense of well-being and have a normal neurologic examination

E. Differential diagnosis of pseudotumor cerebri (Table 9-2)

V.   Optic neuritis

A. Primary inflammation of the optic nerve

B. Two clinical forms of optic neuritis:

      1. Papillitis—intraocular form in which disc swelling is present

      2. Retrobulbar neuritis—optic disc appears normal and inflammatory lesion along course of optic nerve is behind globe

C. Acute impairment of vision

D. Usually unilateral, although may be bilateral, especially in children

E. Occurs in young (14 to 45 years) adults; females outnumber males (5:1)

F. Pain: periocular, retrobulbar, tenderness of the globe, pain especially with eye movement

G. Afferent pupillary defect present if optic neuritis is unilateral

H. Visual field defects: usually central scotoma, but may be centrocecal or nerve fiber bundle defects

I. Cells in vitreous with papillitis

J. Chronological pattern of visual loss: rapid decrease in acuity during the first 2 or 3 days; stable level of decreased vision for 7 to 10 days, then gradual improvement of vision, frequently returning to normal level within 2 to 3 months

K. Uhthoff's symptom: dimming of vision in affected eye with elevation of body temperature (eg, exercise, hot shower, fever) with active or recurrent optic neuritis

L. Etiologies of optic neuritis

      1. Idiopathic

Table 9-2

CONDITIONS ASSOCIATED WITH PSEUDOTUMOR CEREBRI

1. Obstruction or impairment of intracranial venous drainage
   Dural sinus thrombosis
   Radical neck surgery
   Chronic respiratory insufficiency
   Mediastinal mass

2. Endocrine and metabolic dysfunction
Eclampsia	Diabetic ketoacidosis
Hypoparathyroidism	Menarche
Addison's disease	Obesity
Scurvy	Menstrual abnormalities
Oral progestational agents	Pregnancy

3. Exogenously administered agents
Heavy metals: lead, arsenic	Naladixic acid
Vitamin A	Prolonged steroid therapy
Tetracycline	Steroid withdrawal
Amiodarone	Dilantin
Lithium	Amiodarone

4. Systemic illness
   Chronic uremia
   Infectious disease
    Bacterial: subacute bacterial endocarditis (SBE), meningitis
    Viral: meningitis, Guillain-Barré syndrome
    Parasitic: trypanosomiasis, torulosis
    Contiguous infection (middle ear, mastoid)
   Neoplastic disease
    Carcinomatous meningitis
    Leukemia
    Spinal cord tumors
   Hematologic disease
    Hypercoagulable states
    Infectious mononucleosis
    Anemia
    Hemophilia
    Idiopathic thrombocytopenic purpura
   Miscellaneous
    Lupus erythematosus
    Sarcoidosis
    Syphilis
    Paget's disease
    Whipple's disease

2. Multiple sclerosis

3. Viral infections: childhood (eg, mumps, measles, chicken pox), adult (eg, zoster)

4. Postviral syndrome

5. Intraocular inflammation

6. Contiguous inflammation (eg, meninges, orbit, sinuses)

7. Systemic illness (eg, sarcoid, syphilis, tuberculosis)

M. Optic Neuritis Treatment Trial (ONTT)

1. Prospective, randomized study of 457 patients with optic neuritis

2. Three treatment groups:

a. Oral prednisone (1 mg/kg/day) for 14 days

b. Intravenous methylprednisolone (1000 mg/day) for 3 days, followed by oral prednisone (1 g/kg/day) for 11 days

c. Oral placebo for 14 days

3. Fastest recovery for intravenous group, but at 1-year follow-up and thereafter no significant difference in visual recovery among three groups

4. At 1-year follow-up 91% to 95% of patients in three groups regained acuity of 20/40 or better

5. Patients treated with oral prednisone had significantly higher rates of new attacks of optic neuritis

6. Group receiving intravenous regimen and having two or more typical demyelinating white matter lesions on MR scanning; had a significantly lower rate of developing multiple sclerosis within 2 years of follow-up than did the placebo or prednisone groups. However, this benefit was no longer measurable after 3 years of follow-up

7. Visual prognosis for optic neuritis generally good. ONTT at 5 years follow-up:

a. 20/25 or better: 87%

b. 20/30 to 20/40: 7%

c. 20/50 to 20/190: 3%

d. 20/200 or worse: 3%

8. Overall probability of developing clinically definite multiple sclerosis (MS) at 5 years: 30%

9. MRI findings are strongest predictor of developing clinically definite MS at 5-year follow-up:

a. No MRI lesions: 16%

b. Three or more lesions: 51%

VI. **Ischemic optic neuropathy (ION)**

A. Ischemic infarction of the anterior portion of the optic nerve

B. Acute visual loss, usually in patients over the age of 60

C. Clinical settings in which ION is seen

1. Arterial disease

a. Arteritis

i. Giant cell arteritis (Table 9-3)

ii. Collagen diseases

iii. Syphilis

iv. Herpes zoster

Table 9-3

AMERICAN COLLEGE OF RHEUMATOLOGY CRITERIA FOR CLASSIFICATION OF GIANT CELL ARTERITIS

1.   Age at onset of 50 years or older
2.   Onset of new headache
3.   Temporal artery abnormality (tender or reduced pulsation)
4.   Elevated ESR, defined as > 50 mm/hour using Westergren method
5.   Abnormal artery biopsy showing necrotizing vasculitis with predominant mononuclear cell infiltration or granulomatous inflammation

(Sensitivity 93.5%, specificity 91.2% for diagnosis with at least three of five criteria met)

        b. Nonarteritic ischemic optic neuropathy (NAION)—"arteriosclerosis"

        c. Diabetes mellitus

        d. Malignant hypertension

        e. Embolic disease

        f. Vasospastic (migraine)

        g. Post-irradiation

    2. Hypotension/hypovolemia

        a. Massive blood loss

        b. Cardiac insufficiency

        c. Surgical hypotension

        d. Anemia

    3. Other

        a. Post-cataract surgery

        b. Amiodarone

D. Differential diagnosis involves arteritic (giant cell arteritis) versus nonarteritic (arteriosclerotic) as major causes of ischemic optic neuropathy (Table 9-4)

E. ION is virtually always accompanied by disc swelling in the acute stage; rare exception in retrobulbar ischemic optic neuropathy associated with giant cell arteritis

F. Optic disc in NAION is commonly full and cupless ("disc at risk")

G. Visual defect is usually maximal in onset. On occasion, field abnormality may progress within the first month. Subsequent improvement may occur in up to 40% of patients with NAION

H. With arteritic ION, may see marked delay in choroidal perfusion with fluorescein angiography: signifies involvement of posterior ciliary arteries

I. Recognition of cases due to giant cell arteritis is essential; prompt steroid therapy may restore some degree of vision, avert visual loss in the fellow eye, and improve long-term systemic morbidity and mortality

VII. Miscellaneous causes of swollen optic disc

A. Orbital disease

    1. Optic nerve or arachnoid cyst

    2. Orbital tumor

Table 9-4

MAJOR CAUSES OF ISCHEMIC OPTIC NEUROPATHY

	NAION	**Giant Cell Arteritis**
Age peak	60 to 70 years	70 to 80 years
Visual loss	Minimal to severe	Usually severe
Involvement of second eye	Approximately 40%	Approximately 75%
Acute fundus	Swollen disc	Swollen disc, may be pallid
Other ophthalmologic presentations		Central retinal artery occlusion, choroidal infarction, anterior segment ischemia
Systemic	Hypertension (approximately 50%)	Headache, scalp tenderness, malaise, weakness, weight loss, fever, jaw pain, polymyalgia
ESR (Westergren) (mm/hr)	Up to 40	Usually high (50 to 120)
Temporal artery biopsy	May show arteriosclerotic change	Granulomatous inflammation, multinucleated giant cells, disruption of internal elastic lamina
Response to steroids	None	Relief of systemic symptoms, infrequent return to vision, protect other eye

Modified from Glaser JS. Neuro-ophthalmology. In: Duane TD, ed. *Clinical Ophthalmology.* Vol 2. Philadelphia, Pa: Lippincott-Williams & Wilkins; 1994: chapter 5, 55.

3. Dysthyroid optic neuropathy
    a. Unilateral or bilateral progressive visual loss
    b. Patient may have only mild to moderate congestive, orbital signs
    c. Visual field loss typically central scotoma, sometimes combined with inferior depression
    d. Optic disc may appear swollen, normal, or pale
    e. Optic neuropathy due to compression of optic nerve by enlarged extraocular muscles at orbital apex
    f. Treatment: systemic steroids, radiotherapy, orbital decompression surgery

B. Intraocular disease: uveitis, vein occlusion, disc tumor, hypotony

C. Diabetic papillopathy (diabetic papillitis, "acute disc swelling in juvenile diabetes")
    1. Onset: second to eighth decades (average: 50 years)
    2. Type I or II diabetics of some chronicity (average: 10 to 12 years)
    3. Commonly bilateral but may be unilateral
    4. Disc edema with prominent telangiectatic change without neovascularization

5. No correlation with degree of diabetic retinopathy
6. Frequently asymptomatic or modest acuity loss to 20/50; occasionally more profound loss
7. Visual field defects include enlarged blind spot and arcuate defects
8. Generally good visual prognosis with return of normal acuity in 3 months to 1 year
9. Visual improvement precedes disappearance of disc swelling
10. Disc usually regains normal appearance, although may also develop diffuse or segmental pallor

D. Papillophlebitis (retinal vasculitis, optic disc vasculitis, "big blind spot syndrome")
   1. Usually unilateral disc edema
   2. Young, healthy adults
   3. Vague visual complaints of blurred vision with minimal impairment of acuity (usually no worse than 20/30)
   4. No afferent pupillary defect
   5. Only visual field abnormality is enlargement of blind spot
   6. Disc swelling with associated engorged retinal veins and occasional retinal hemorrhages
   7. Spontaneous, usually complete recovery within several months to 1 year
   8. Pathologic examination reveals inflammation of the retinal veins, although etiology of inflammation is unknown
   9. Rarely, "big blind spot syndrome" seen without optic disc edema
      a. Often accompanied with subjective photopsias in area of blind spot
      b. May be associated with retinal disorder such as multiple evanescent white dot syndrome (MEWDS)
      c. Benign, self-limited clinical cause
      d. Etiology: transient peripapillary photoreceptor dysfunction of unknown cause

E. Leber's hereditary optic neuropathy (see Table 10-1)
   1. Most often, but not exclusively, affects males in the second or third decade of life
   2. Rapid monocular visual loss to a variable level (20/200 or worse)
   3. Second eye usually affected within days or weeks
   4. In acute phase, optic disc may appear normal or have typical triad of findings
      a. Circumpapillary telangiectatic microangiopathy
      b. Prominent nerve fiber layer around disc
      c. Absence of dye leakage from the disc or peripapillary region with fluorescein angiography
   5. Visual field abnormality is centrocecal scotoma
   6. Ultimately, the patient develops either temporal or generalized disc pallor
   7. Maternal inheritance pattern in Leber's hereditary optic neuropathy
      a. Disorder of mitochondrial, not chromosomal, DNA
      b. Chromosomal DNA follows Mendelian pattern of inheritance, but mitochondrial DNA is inherited exclusively from the mother
      c. Leber's optic neuropathy linked with several point mutations in mitochondrial DNA, most commonly 11778, but also 14484, 3460
      d. Mitochondrial DNA is essential for oxydative phosphorylation, the energy-producing cycle in the cell

       e. Heteroplasmy: intracellular mitochondrial DNA is a mixture of mutant and normal forms; provides basis for variable clinical expression of mutation

   8. EKG obtained to exclude potential cardiac conduction defect

   9. No effective treatment—eliminate use of tobacco, alcohol

F. Spheno-orbital meningioma

   1. Chronic compression of the intraorbital or intracanalicular optic nerve

   2. Clinical triad

       a. Visual loss

       b. Optic disc swelling that resolves into optic atrophy

       c. Appearance of optociliary shunt vessels

   3. The clinical picture may also be seen with optic nerve glioma, chronic papilledema, craniopharyngioma

G. Optic disc edema with macular star

   1. Descriptive term that includes several different disease processes

   2. Main clinical settings:

       a. Inflammatory papillitis

       b. Vascular disorders (hypertension, diabetes mellitus)

       c. Papilledema

       d. Infectious/immune mediated

   3. Neuroretinitis is a general description often applied to infectious/immune-mediated cause

   4. Leber's idiopathic stellate neuroretinitis

       a. Triad: visual loss, optic disc edema, macular star

       b. Children and young adults

       c. Antecedent viral illness in up to 50% of patients

       d. Generally benign, self-limited condition

       e. Resolution of disc edema in 3 months; up to 1 year for macular star to resolve

       f. Visual prognosis usually good

   5. Neuroretinitis may be due to organisms other than virus:

       a. Cat scratch disease (Bartonella henselae)

       b. Toxoplasmosis

       c. Toxocariasis

       d. Histoplasmosis

       e. Spirochetoses (syphilis, Lyme disease)

VIII. Pseudopapilledema (anomalous elevation of the disc; congenitally full disc)

A. Ophthalmoscopic features

   1. Disc is not hyperemic, and there are no dilated capillaries on its surface

   2. Despite disc elevation, surface arteries are not obscured (no peripapillary nerve fiber layer opacification)

   3. Physiologic cup usually absent

   4. May see anomalous branching and tortuosity of retinal vessels (abnormally large number of branches at disc margin)

   5. May see drusen (hyaline bodies) buried in disc of patient or relatives

   6. No hemorrhages (rare exceptions)

7. No exudates or cotton-wool spots
8. Disc usually has irregular border with pigment epithelial defects in peripapillary retina
9. Visual field testing may show enlarged blind spots and nerve fiber bundle defects

B. If exam is suggestive of buried disc drusen, may use orbital ultrasonography or CT to "visualize" them

BIBLIOGRAPHY

Books

Kline LB, ed. Optic nerve disorders. *Ophthalmology Monographs.* Vol 10. San Francisco, Calif: American Academy of Ophthalmology; 1996.

Spoor TC. *Atlas of Optic Nerve Disorders.* New York, NY: Raven Press; 1992.

Chapters

Glaser JS. Topical diagnosis: prechiasmal visual pathway. In: Duane TD, ed. *Clinical Ophthalmology.* Vol 2. Philadelphia, Pa: Lippincott-Williams & Wilkins; 1998: chapter 5, 1-85.

Martin TJ, Corbett JJ. *Neuro-ophthalmology—The Requisites.* St. Louis, Mo: Mosby; 2000: 57-94.

Articles

Appen RE, de Venecia G, Ferwerda J. Optic disc vasculitis. *Am J Ophthalmol.* 1980;90:352-359.

Barr CC, Glaser JS, Blankenship G. Acute disc swelling in juvenile diabetes. Clinical profile and natural history of 12 cases. *Arch Ophthalmol.* 1980; 92:2185-2192.

Beck RW, Cleary PA. The optic neuritis treatment trial: three-year follow-up results. *Arch Ophthalmol.* 1995;113:136.

Beck RW, Cleary PA, Optic Neuritis Study Group. Optic Neuritis Treatment Trial: one-year follow-up results. *Arch Ophthalmol.* 1993;111:773-775.

Beck RW, Cleary PA, Trobe JD, et al. The effect of corticosteroids for acute optic neuritis on the subsequent development of multiple sclerosis. *N Engl J Med.* 1993;329:1764-1769.

Boghen DR, Glaser JS. Ischemic optic neuropathy. The clinical profile and natural history. *Brain.* 1975;98:689-708.

Carter KD, Frueh BR, Hessburg TP, et al. Long-term efficacy of orbital decompression for compressive optic neuropathy of Graves' eye disease. *Ophthalmology.* 1991;98:1435-1442.

Cogan DG. Blackouts not obviously due to carotid occlusion. *Arch Ophthalmol.* 1961;66:180-187.

Corbett JJ, Savino PJ, Thompson HS, et al. Visual loss in pseudotumor cerebri. Follow-up of 57 patients from five to 41 years and a profile of 14 patients with permanent severe visual loss. *Arch Neurol.* 1982;39:461-474.

Dreyer RF, Hopen G, Gass JD, Smith JL. Leber's idiopathic stellate neuroretinitis. *Arch Ophthalmol.* 1984;102:1140-1145.

Fletcher WA. The big blind spot syndromes. *Ophthalmol Clin NA.* 1991;4:531-546.

Frisén L, Hoyt WF, Tengroth BM. Optociliary veins, disc pallor, and visual loss: a triad of signs indicating spheno-orbital meningioma. *Acta Ophthalmol.* 1973;51:241-249.

Hayreh MS, Hayreh SS. Optic disc edema in raised intracranial pressure: I. Evaluation and resolution. *Arch Ophthalmol.* 1977;95:1237-1244.

Hayreh MS, Hayreh SS. Optic disc edema in raised intracranial pressure: II. Early detection with fluorescein fundus angiography and stereoscopic color photography. *Arch Ophthalmol.* 1977;95:1245-1254.

Hayreh SS. Optic disc edema in raised intracranial pressure: V. Pathogenesis. *Arch Ophthalmol.* 1977;95:1553-1565.

Hayreh SS. Optic disc edema in raised intracranial pressure: VI. Associated visual disturbances and their pathogenesis. *Arch Ophthalmol.* 1977;95:1566-1579.

Levin BE. The clinical significance of spontaneous pulsations of the retinal vein. *Arch Neurol.* 1978;35:37-40.

Lonn LI, Hoyt WF. Papillophlebitis: a cause of protracted yet benign optic disc edema. *Eye Ear Nose Throat Monthly.* 1966;45:62-68.

Miller GR, Smith JL. Ischemic optic neuropathy. *Am J Ophthalmol.* 1966;62:103-115.

Minkler DS, Tso MOM, Zimmerman LE. A light microscopic, autoradiographic study of axoplasmic transport in the optic nerve head during ocular hypotony, increased intracranial pressure, and papilledema. *Am J Ophthalmol.* 1976;82:741-759.

Newman NJ. Leber's hereditary optic neuropathy. *Ophthalmol Clin NA.* 1991;4:431-447.

Okun E. Chronic papilledema simulating hyaline bodies of the optic disc. *Am J Ophthalmol.* 1962;53:922-927.

Regillo CP, Brown GC, Savino PJ, et al. Diabetic papillopathy. *Arch Ophthalmol.* 1995;113:889-895.

Rizzo JF, Lessell S. Risk of developing multiple sclerosis after uncomplicated optic neuritis. *Neurology.* 1988;38:185-190.

Rosenberg MA, Savino PJ, Glaser JS. A clinical analysis of pseudopapilledema: I. Population, laterality, acuity, refractive error, ophthalmoscopic characteristics, and coincident disease. *Arch Ophthalmol.* 1979;97:65-70.

Rush JA. Pseudotumor cerebri: clinical profile and visual outcome in 63 patients. *Mayo Clin Proc.* 1980;55:541-546.

Savino PJ, Glaser JS, Rosenburg MA. A clinical analysis of pseudopapilledema: II. Visual field defects. *Arch Ophthalmol.* 1979;97:71-75.

Smith JL, Hoyt WF, Susac JO. Ocular fundus in acute Leber's optic neuropathy. *Arch Ophthalmol.* 1973;90:349-354.

Solley A, Martin DF, Newman NJ. Cat scratch disease. Posterior segment manifestation. *Ophthalmology.* 1999;106:1546-1553.

Spencer WH. Drusen of the optic disc and aberrant axoplasmic transport. The XXIII Edward Jackson Memorial Lecture. *Am J Ophthalmol.* 1978;85:1-12.

The Ischemic Optic Neuropathy Decompression Trial Research Group. Optic nerve decompression surgery for nonarteritic ischemic optic neuropathy is not effective and may be harmful. *JAMA.* 1995;273:625-632.

The Optic Neuritis Study Group. The 5-year risk of MS after optic neuritis: experience of the Optic Neuritis Treatment Trial. *Neurology.* 1997;49:1404-1413.

The Optic Neuritis Study Group. Visual function 5 years after optic neuritis: experience of the Optic Neuritis Treatment Trial. *Arch Ophthalmol.* 1997;115:1545-1552.

Tso MO, Hayreh SS. Optic disc edema in raised intracranial pressure: III. A pathologic study of experimental papilledema. *Arch Ophthalmol.* 1977;95:1448-1457.

Tso MO, Hayreh SS. Optic disc edema in raised intracranial pressure: IV. Axoplasmic transport in experimental papilledema. *Arch Ophthalmol.* 1977;95:1458-1462.

Chapter 10

The Pale Optic Disc: Optic Atrophy

I. **Optic disc pallor versus optic atrophy**

A. Ophthalmoscopic appearance of disc pallor alone does not establish the presence of optic atrophy

B. Frequently, the temporal side of the normal disc has less color than the nasal side

C. Optic atrophy is a pathologic description of optic nerve shrinkage from any process that produces degeneration of axons in the anterior visual system (retinogeniculate) pathway

D. The clinical diagnosis of optic atrophy is based on:
   1. Ophthalmoscopic abnormalities of color and structure of the disc with associated changes in retinal vessels and nerve fiber layer
   2. Defective visual function (acuity, color vision pupils, fields, visual evoked response) and can be localized to the optic nerve

II. **Histopathologic considerations**

A. When a visual axon is severed, its ascending (to the brain) segment disintegrates and disappears in approximately 7 days. This is termed Wallerian degeneration

B. The portion of the axon still connected to the ganglion cell body remains viable for 3 to 4 weeks but then rapidly degenerates by 6 to 8 weeks. This is called descending (to the eye) degeneration

C. With the completion of descending degeneration of axons, optic disc pallor appears. Currently, there are two major theories to explain acquired disc pallor
   1. Vascular-glial theory: when the optic nerve degenerates, its blood supply is reduced and smaller vessels, recognizable in the normal disc, disappear from view. In addition, formation of glial tissue at the nerve head is said to occur with optic atrophy
   2. Nerve fiber layer theory (Figure 10-1): with degeneration of visual axons, there is alteration in the thickness and cytoarchitecture of nerve fiber bundles passing between glial columns containing capillaries. Alteration of light conducted along the nerve fiber bundles leads to the appearance of pallor, and there is no reduction in blood supply to the optic disc

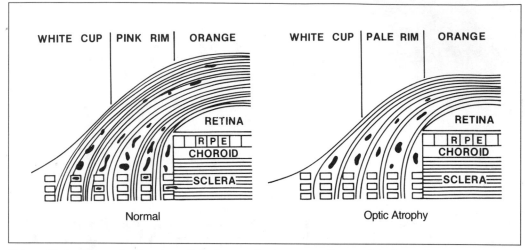

Figure 10-1. Schematic drawing of the longitudinal section of normal and atrophic optic discs. In optic atrophy, there is a decrease in the number of nerve fibers and capillaries, but the proportion of capillaries per unit volume is unchanged (modified from Quigley HA, Anderson DR. The histologic basis of optic disc pallor in experimental optic atrophy. *Am J Ophthalmol.* 1977;83:709-717).

III. Ophthalmoscopic features of optic atrophy

A. As a general rule, fundus signs are not specific for any particular etiology of optic atrophy, and the diagnosis must be obtained from nonophthalmoscopic findings

B. In the early stages of atrophy, the optic disc loses its reddish hue, and the substance of the disc slowly melts away to leave a pale, shallow concave meniscus—the exposed lamina cribrosa

C. Ipsilateral attenuation of the retinal arterioles is frequently a sign of old central retinal artery occlusion

D. Healed papillitis or ischemic optic neuropathy may cause narrowing of retinal arterioles only in their peripapillary segment, after which they appear to enlarge slightly in caliber as they traverse the fundus ("reverse taper sign")

E. Pathologic disc cupping may develop, along with disc pallor, in patients without glaucoma. Etiologies include ischemia, compression, inflammation, and trauma

F. Nerve fiber layer defects should be carefully looked for when suspecting optic atrophy. They appear as dark slits or wedges and are most easily identified in the superior and inferior arcuate regions where the nerve fiber layer is particularly thick. Also, vessels in this area, having lost their surrounding nerve fiber covering, appear darker than normal and stand out sharply

G. "Bow-tie" or "band" optic atrophy (Figure 10-2)
   1. Specific patterns of nerve fiber layer and optic atrophy from optic chiasmal and retrochiasmal-pregeniculate lesions
   2. With temporal field defects, loss of nerve fiber from ganglion cells nasal to fovea
   3. Results in atrophy of nasal and temporal portions of the disc, with relative sparing of superior and inferior arcuate bundles

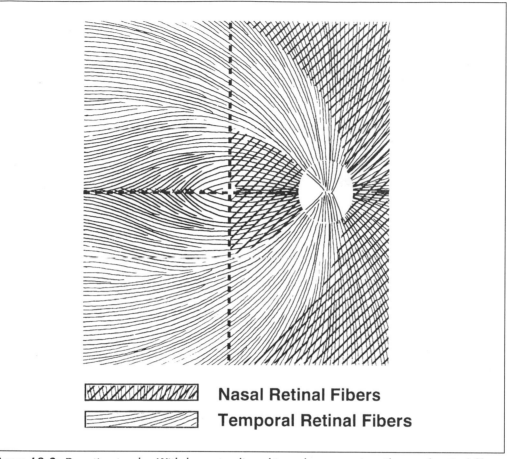

Nasal Retinal Fibers
Temporal Retinal Fibers

Figure 10-2. Bow-tie atrophy. With long-standing chiasmal compression, the nasal retinal fibers become atrophic, and pallor is seen in a pattern corresponding to the location of the fibers in the optic disc (modified from Newman NJ. Chiasm, parachiasmal syndromes, retrochiasm and disorders of higher visual function. In: Slamovits TL, Burde RM, eds. *Neuro-ophthalmology.* St. Louis, Mo: Mosby-Year Book; 1994:4-7).

  4. Arcuate bundles are spared since they arise from ganglion cells both temporal and nasal to the fovea

H. Optic nerve hypoplasia
  1. Incomplete development of the optic nerve
  2. Unilateral or bilateral
  3. Variable acuity depending upon degree of development
  4. Double ring sign: hypoplastic disc surrounded by ring of sclera and ring of hyperpigmentation
  5. Clinical settings:
    a. Unilateral: isolated or accompanied by strabismus and/or nystagmus
    b. Bilateral: forebrain malformation and endocrinologic defects
      i. Septo-optic dysplasia (de Morsier's syndrome)

        ii. Short stature

        iii. Absence of septum pellucidum

        iv. Endocrine deficits: growth hormone, hypothyroidism, sexual development, diabetes insipidus

    6. Associated conditions

        a. Maternal diabetes mellitus

        b. Fetal alcohol syndrome

        c. Use of LSD, quinine, antiepileptic drugs during pregnancy

    7. Patient evaluation (bilateral cases)

        a. Cranial magnetic resonance imaging (MRI)

        b. Endocrinologic and neurologic evaluations

  I. Homonymous hemioptic hypoplasia

    1. Optic disc findings in patients with congenital cerebral hemiatrophy, presumably due to fetal vascular insufficiency

    2. Fundus ipsilateral to hemispheric defect shows slightly small optic disc with temporal pallor and loss of nerve fiber layer of ganglion cells temporal to the fovea

    3. Fundus contralateral to hemispheric defect shows small disc with "band" atrophy

    4. Associated findings include mental retardation, seizures, congenital hemiplegia, and complete homonymous hemianopia

IV. The hereditary optic neuropathies

A. These forms of optic nerve disease often cause insidious, bilateral, symmetric loss of central acuity

B. Table 10-1 summarizes the major forms of hereditary optic nerve disease

V. Toxic and deficiency optic neuropathies

A. Particular forms of medical therapy or exposure to specific toxins may lead to bilateral retrobulbar optic neuropathy, characterized by visual loss, severe dyschromatopsia, central field defects with occasional peripheral field constriction, and initially normal-appearing optic discs that may gradually become pale

B. Frequently used drugs that may cause optic atrophy include:

    1. Ethambutol

    2. Isoniazid

    3. Chloramphenicol

    4. Streptomycin

    5. Digitalis

    6. Chloroquine

    7. Placidyl

    8. Chlorpropamide

    9. Rifampin

C. *Grant's Toxicology of the Eye* lists over 20 toxins associated with optic neuropathy, including:

    1. Arsenic

    2. Lead

Table 10-1

HEREDOFAMILIAL OPTIC ATROPHIES

| | Disorders of Chromosomal DNA | | | | Disorder of Mitochondrial DNA |
	Dominant Juvenile (infantile)	Early infantile (congenital); simple	Recessive Behr's type; complicated	With diabetes mellitus; ± deafness	Maternal Leber's disease
Age at onset	Childhood (4 to 8 years)	Early childhood* (3 to 4 years)	Childhood (1 to 9 years)	Childhood (6 to 14 years)	Early adulthood (18 to 30 years; up to sixth decade)
Visual impairment	Mild/moderate (20/40 - 20/200)	Severe (20/200 - HM)	Moderate (20/200)	Severe (20/400 - FC)	Moderate/severe (20/200 - FC)
Nystagmus	Rare†	Usual	In 50%	Absent	Absent
Optic disc	Mild temporal pallor; ± temporal excavation	Marked diffuse pallor (± arteriolar attenuation)‡	Mild temporal pallor	Marked diffuse pallor	Moderate diffuse pallor; disc swelling in acute phase
Color vision	Blue-yellow dyschromatopsia	Severe dyschromatopsia/ achromatopsia	Moderate to severe dyschromatopsia	Severe cyschromatopsia	Dense central scotoma for colors
Course	Variable; slight progression	Stable	Stable	Progressive	Acute visual loss, then usually stable; may improve/worsen

HM = hand motions; FC = finger counting

*Difficult to assess in infancy, but visual impairment usually manifests by age 4 years

†Presence of nystagmus with poor vision and earlier onset suggests separate congenital or infantile form

‡Distinguished from tapetoretinal degenerations by normal electroretinogram (ERG)

Modified from Glaser JS. Heredofamilial disorders of the optic nerve. In: Renie WA, ed. *Goldberg's Genetic and Metabolic Eye Disease.* 2nd ed. Boston, Mass: Little, Brown & Co; 1986: chapter 18, p. 471.

      3. Hexachlorophene (PhisoHex)

      4. Methanol

      5. Lysol

      6. Quinine

      7. Ethylene glycol

D. Deficiency optic neuropathies

      1. Clinical picture of progressive bilateral visual loss, with central or centrocecal scotomas and some degree of temporal disc pallor and atrophy of the papillomacular nerve fiber layer

      2. Vitamin deficiencies that may be responsible for optic atrophy include:

         a Vitamin B_{12} (cobalamin)

         b. Vitamin B_6 (pyridoxine)

         c. Vitamin B_1 (thiamine)

         d. Niacin

         e. Vitamin B_2 (riboflavin)

         f. Folic acid

E. Tobacco-alcohol amblyopia

      1. Similar clinical picture to deficiency optic neuropathies listed above

      2. Continuing controversy as to whether this represents a form of toxic (cyanide) or deficiency (vitamin) optic nerve disease

      3. In general, prognosis for recovery of vision is good except in the most chronic cases

VI. Primary optic nerve neoplasms

A. Optic glioma

      1. Two major forms: childhood (benign) and adulthood (malignant) (Table 10-2)

      2. Childhood form

         a. Patient presents with visual loss, proptosis, occasionally monocular nystagmus ("spasmus nutans," see Chapter 3)

         b. One/both optic nerves and/or chiasm

         c. Up to 25% may have neurofibromatosis

         d. Neuroimaging: double-intensity tubular thickening and kinking of orbital optic nerve(s), enlargement of chiasm, infiltration of hypothalamus

         e. Treatment controversial: surgery, radiation therapy, chemotherapy

      3. Adult form

         a. Rapid onset of visual loss and relentless deterioration

         b. Usually begins in chiasm

         c. Neuroimaging: suprasellar mass with edema

         d. Treatment: radiation only palliative

B. Optic nerve sheath meningioma

      1. Typically occurs in young to middle-aged women

      2. Insidious, progressive visual loss

      3. Most commonly unilateral, but may be bilateral

      4. Associated with neurofibromatosis

      5. Optic disc chronically swollen, becomes pale, with appearance of optociliary shunt vessels

Table 10-2		
PRIMARY GLIOMAS OF THE OPTIC NERVE AND CHIASM		
	Childhood	**Adulthood**
Age at onset of symptoms	4 to 8 years	Middle age
Presentation	Visual loss, proptosis	Rapid severe visual loss
Course	Relatively stable, nonprogressive	Rapid bilateral visual deterioration, other intracranial signs (eg, confusion, lethargy)
Prognosis	Compatible with long life	Death within months to 2 years
Neurofibromatosis	Associated in up to 25% of cases	No relationship
Histology	Pilocystic astrocytoma	Malignant astrocytoma (glioblastoma)

Modified from Glaser JS. *Neuro-ophthalmology.* Hagerstown, Md: Harper & Row; 1978: 117.

      6. Neuroimaging

          a. Computed tomography (CT): "tram-track" appearance due to calcification

          b. MRI: enhancement, able to detect intracranial spread through optic canal

      7. Treatment: radiation therapy; surgery with evidence of intracranial progression

VII. Infiltrative optic neuropathy

A. Optic disc initially swollen or normal; ultimately becomes pale

B. Often acute visual loss

C. Etiology may be benign or malignant

    1. Sarcoidosis

    2. Lymphoma

    3. Leukemia

    4. Plasmacytoma

    5. Malignant histiocytosis

VIII. Carcinomatous optic neuropathy

A. Fundus typically normal at onset of visual loss, with disc gradually becoming pale

B. Patient may or may not have history of known malignancy

C. Optic neuropathy may be isolated or accompanied by other neurologic defects

D. Visual loss typically acute and devastating

E. Unless large intraparenchymal central nervous system (CNS) spread has occurred, radiologic studies (CT, MRI, angiography) are often normal

F. May see meningeal enhancement with cranial MR scanning following IV contrast

G. Careful cerebrospinal fluid (CSF) analysis with cytologic examination for malignant cells

H. Due to microscopic infiltrates of the nerve and its sheaths

IX. Radiation optic neuropathy

A. Due to delayed radionecrosis of optic nerve and chiasm

B. Follows radiation therapy (external beam, gamma knife) for perisellar tumor, such as pituitary adenoma, craniopharyngioma, invasive sinus carcinoma

C. Diagnostic criteria
   1. Acute visual loss (monocular or binocular)
   2. Visual field defects indicating optic nerve or chiasmal dysfunction
   3. Optic disc edema usually absent (Chapter 9, Section VI)
   4. Onset usually within 3 years of therapy (peak: 1 to 1.5 years)
   5. Neuroimaging studies demonstrate no evidence of anterior visual pathway compression
   6. Contrast-enhanced MR scanning may demonstrate areas of increased signal in optic nerves and/or chiasm

D. Pathology: fibrinoid necrosis of blood vessels, demyelination, necrosis

E. Treatment: none of proven efficacy

X. Traumatic optic neuropathy

A. Three categories:
   1. Evulsion
   2. Direct injury
   3. Indirect injury

B. Optic nerve evulsion
   1. Dislocation of optic nerve from scleral canal
   2. Partial or complete
   3. As early vitreous hemorrhage clears optic disc partially or totally absent
   4. May be confirmed with imaging studies (ultrasound, CT, MRI)
   5. Treatment: none

C. Direct injury
   1. Impact on optic nerve or its sheaths by a blunt or sharp object
   2. With anterior injury, may see fundus picture of central retinal artery occlusion (CRAO)
   3. More posterior involvement leads to normal fundus appearance followed by optic atrophy within 4 to 8 weeks
   4. Multiple pathophysiologic mechanisms
      a. Laceration
      b. Bone deformation/fracture
      c. Vascular insufficiency
      d. Hemorrhage
   5. Imaging studies: CT, MRI (contraindicated with ferromagnetic foreign body)
   6. Treatment individualized; megadose IV steroids, surgery

D. Indirect injury
   1. Blunt trauma to orbit or cranium with lines of force transmitted to orbital apex
   2. Most common form of traumatic optic neuropathy
   3. Canalicular optic nerve is site of injury

4. Fundus initially normal with appearance of optic atrophy in 4 to 8 weeks
5. Imaging studies may be normal or demonstrate optic canal fracture
6. Pathophysiologic mechanisms, as with direct injury (see above)
7. Treatment: none of proven efficacy

BIBLIOGRAPHY

Books

Kline LB, ed. Optic nerve disorders. *Ophthalmology Monographs.* Vol 10. San Francisco, Calif: American Academy of Ophthalmology; 1996.

Spoor TC. *Atlas of Optic Nerve Disorders.* New York, NY: Raven Press; 1992.

Chapters

Glaser JS. Heredofamilial disorders of the optic nerve. In: Goldberg MF, ed. *Genetic and Metabolic Eye Disease.* 2nd ed. Boston, Mass: Little, Brown & Co; 1974: 463-486.

Articles

Dutton JJ. Gliomas of the anterior visual pathway. *Surv Ophthalmol.* 1994;38:427-452.

Dutton JJ. Optic nerve sheath meningiomas. *Surv Ophthalmol.* 1992;37:167-183.

Eibert H, Kjer B, Kjer P, et al. Dominant optic atrophy mapped to chromosome 3q region I. Linage analysis. *Human Mol Genet.* 1994;3:977-980.

Eng TY, Albright NW, Kuwahara G, et al. Precision radiation therapy for optic nerve sheath meningiomas. *Int J Radiat Oncol Biol Phys.* 1992;22:1093-1098.

Haik BG, Saint Louis L, Bierly J, et al. Magnetic resonance imaging in the evaluation of optic nerve gliomas. *Ophthalmology.* 1997;94:709-717.

Hoyt WF, Rios-Montenegro EN, Behrens MM, et al. Homonymous hemioptic hypoplasia: funduscopic features in standard and red-free illumination in three patients with congenital hemiplegia. *Br J Ophthalmol.* 1972;56:537-545.

Hoyt WF, Baghdassarian SA. Optic glioma of childhood: natural history and rationale for conservative management. *Br J Ophthalmol.* 1969;53:793-798.

Hoyt WF, Meshal LG, Lessell S, et al. Malignant optic glioma of adulthood. *Brain.* 1973;96:121-132.

Imes RK, Hoyt WF. Childhood chiasmal gliomas: update on the fate of patients in the 1969 San Francisco study. *Br J Ophthalmol.* 1986;70:179-182.

Kline LB, Glaser JS. Dominant optic atrophy: the clinical profile. *Arch Ophthalmol.* 1979;97:1680-1686.

Kline LB, Kim JY, Ceballos R. Radiation optic neuropathy. *Ophthalmology.* 1985,92:1118-1126.

Lambert SR, Hoyt CS, Narahara MH. Optic nerve hypoplasia. *Surv Ophthalmol.* 1987;32:1-9.

Lessell S, Gise RL, Krohel GB. Bilateral optic neuropathy with remission in young man. Variation on a theme by Leber? *Arch Neurol.* 1983;40:2-6.

Levin LA, Beck RW, Joseph JP. The treatment of traumatic optic neuropathy: the international optic nerve trauma study. *Ophthalmology.* 1999;106:1268-1277.

Lindblom B, Truwit CL, Hoyt WF. Optic nerve sheath meningioma; definition of intraorbital intracanalicular, and intracranial components with magnetic resonance imaging. *Ophthalmology.* 1992;99:560-566.

Nikoskelainen E, Hoyt WF, Nummelin K. Ophthalmologic findings in Leber's hereditary optic neuropathy: I. Fundus findings in asymptomatic family members. *Arch Ophthalmol.* 1982;100:1597-1602.

Nikoskelainen E, Hoyt WF, Nummelin K. Ophthalmologic findings in Leber's hereditary optic neuropathy: II. The fundus findings in the affected family member. *Arch Ophthalmol.* 1983;101:1059-1060.

Nikoskelainen E, Hoyt WF, Nummelin K, et al. Ophthalmologic findings in Leber's hereditary optic neuropath, III. Fluorescein angiographic studies. *Arch Ophthalmol.* 1984;102:981-989.

Steinsapir KD, Goldberg RA. Traumatic optic neuropathy. *Surv Ophthalmol.* 1994;38:487-518.

Trobe JD, Glaser JS, Cassady JC. Optic atrophy. Differential diagnosis by fundus observation alone. *Arch Ophthalmol.* 1980;98:1040-1045.

Trobe JD, Glaser JS, Cassady JC, et al. Nonglaucomatous excavation of the optic disc. *Arch Ophthalmol.* 1980;98:1046-1050.

Unsöld R, Hoyt WF. Band atrophy of the optic nerve. The histology of temporal hemianopsia. *Arch Ophthalmol.* 1980;98:1637-1638.

Victor M. Tobacco alcohol amblyopia: a critique of current concepts of this disorder, with special reference to the role of nutritional deficiency in its causation. *Arch Ophthalmol.* 1963;70:313-318.

Zimmerman CF, Schatz NJ, Glaser JS. Magnetic resonance imaging of radiation optic neuropathy. *Am J Ophthalmol.* 1990;110:389-394.

Chapter 11

Myasthenia and Ocular Myopathies

I. **Myasthenia and ocular myopathies**

    A. These disorders produce ocular motor dysfunction due to involvement of the extraocular muscles and the neuromuscular junction

    B. Some of these entities may simulate isolated or combined ocular motor cranial nerve palsies

II. **Myasthenia gravis**

    A. Disease characterized clinically by muscle weakness and fatigue

    B. It is the most common disorder affecting the neuromuscular junction

    C. Myasthenia involves skeletal and not visceral musculature; therefore, the pupil and ciliary muscle are unaffected. Major ophthalmologic complaints are ptosis and diplopia

    D. Ocular involvement eventually occurs in 90% of myasthenics and accounts for the initial complaint in 75%. Approximately 80% of patients with ocular onset progress to involvement of other muscle groups (usually within 2 years), while 20% have only ocular complaints

    E. Impaired neuromuscular transmission of myasthenia is due to the presence of antibodies to acetylcholine receptors in the motor endplate of striated muscles. This leads to a reduction in the number of acetylcholine receptors

    F. Clinical characteristics of ocular myasthenia:

        1. Variability of muscle function within minutes, hours, days, or weeks

        2. Remissions and exacerbations (often triggered by infection or trauma)

        3. Onset at any age

        4. Ptosis (unilateral or bilateral) worse at end of day, may "shift" from eye to eye

        5. Extraocular muscle involvement follows no set pattern; any ocular movement pattern may develop and thus mimic any ocular motor cranial nerve palsy or central gaze disturbance (eg, gaze palsy, INO, gaze-evoked nystagmus)

        6. Dysthyroidism is found in approximately 5% of myasthenics, also an increased incidence of thymoma and collagen vascular disorders

G. Diagnosis of ocular myasthenia
1. Lid fatigue: with sustained upward gaze ptosis, becomes more marked
2. Lid-twitch sign (Cogan): the patient looks down for 10 to 15 seconds and is then asked to rapidly refixate in the primary position. A positive lid-twitch sign consists of an upward overshoot of the lid, which then falls to its previously ptotic position
3. Enhanced ptosis: if ptosis is asymmetric, the patient may use the frontalis muscle to elevate both lids, producing what appears to be lid retraction on one side. If the more ptotic lid is elevated, the previously retracted one will fall
4. Variability in measuring phorias or tropias during the same examination or at different times is very suggestive of myasthenia
5. Myasthenic ptosis is frequently associated with orbicularis weakness
6. Tensilon (edrophonium chloride) test: one positive test establishes the diagnosis of myasthenia, yet myasthenia may exist even in the face of a negative Tensilon test (see Chapter 20 for correct way to perform a Tensilon test)
7. **Alert!** Rarely:
    a. Patient may have false-positive Tensilon test, or
    b. Positive Tensilon test and coexistent intracranial mass (patient has two diseases)
8. Sleep test
    a. Safe alternative to Tensilon test
    b. Resolution of ptosis or ophthalmoparesis after 30-minute period of sleep, with reappearance of sign 30 seconds to 5 minutes after awakening
9. Ice test
    a. Also safe alternative to Tensilon test
    b. Resolution of ptosis after 2-minute application of ice pack to involved eyelid
    c. High degree of sensitivity and specificity for myasthenic ptosis
10. Acetylcholine receptor antibodies, if present, are diagnostic of myasthenia. However, only about one-third of patients with ocular myasthenia have detectable antibody levels
11. Electromyography (EMG): with repetitive supramaximal motor nerve stimulation there is a decremental muscular response in myasthenia. Helpful if present, but may be a normal response in clinically uninvolved extremity musculature in patients with ocular myasthenia. Should be performed on orbicularis oculi as well

H. Certain drugs may cause:
1. Unmasking or aggravation of myasthenia (eg, quinidine, propranolol, lithium)
2. Drug-induced myasthenia syndrome (eg, penicillamine)

I. Treatment of ocular myasthenia
1. Occlusion of one eye
2. Prism spectacles
3. Pyridostigmine (Mestinon)
4. Systemic steroids

J. Treatment of systemic myasthenia
1. Pyridostigmine (Mestinon)
2. Immunosuppressants (steroids, cyclosporine, azathioprine)
3. Plasmaphresis

4. IV immune globulin (IG)

5. Thymectomy

III.   Chronic progressive external ophthalmoplegia (CPEO)

A. Comprises a group of disorders characterized by insidiously progressive, symmetric immobility of the eyes, with lids typically ptotic, the orbicularis oculi weak, and the pupils spared

B. The eye movements remain limited with doll's head and caloric stimulation

C. CPEO may occur in an isolated ocular form, may have a hereditary pattern, or may be part of a recognizable clinical entity

    1. Oculopharyngeal dystrophy: dysphagia, family history of ophthalmoplegia, often of French-Canadian ancestry

    2. Kearns-Sayre syndrome: triad of CPEO, cardiac conduction defect, pigmentary retinopathy

    3. Ophthalmoplegia plus: term applied to instances in which CPEO is associated with the above abnormalities *plus* a variety of others, including elevated cerebrospinal fluid (CSF) protein, spongiform degeneration of the cerebrum and brainstem, slow EEG, subnormal intelligence, hearing loss

D. Muscle biopsy (ocular or limb) will demonstrate mitochondrial accumulations beneath the plasma membrane and between myofibrils. Using a modified trichrome stain, these abnormal muscle fibers have been called "ragged red" fibers

E. CPEO in itself or as part of a multisystem disease may be associated with deletions in the mitochondrial DNA of skeletal muscle ("mitochondrial myopathy")

F. A condition simulating CPEO is known as progressive supranuclear palsy (PSP) or Steele-Richardson-Olszewski syndrome

    1. Vertical gaze, especially downward gaze, is affected first

    2. Eventually horizontal gaze is involved

    3. Doll's head and caloric testing demonstrate full excursions until late in course of disease

    4. Additional clinical findings: dystonic rigidity of neck and trunk, masked face, dysesthesia, hyperreflexia, dementia, apraxia of eyelid opening

    5. Neurodegenerative condition characterized pathologically by neuronal loss, gliosis, neurofibrillary tangles, and demyelination centered in the brainstem reticular formation and ocular motor nuclei

IV.   Myotonic dystrophy

A. Autosomal dominant muscular dystrophy in which myotonia is accompanied by dystrophic changes in other tissues and organs

B. Myotonia is a phenomenon in which muscle fibers have a pathologically persistent activity after a strong contraction or are continuously active when they should be relaxed

C. Ophthalmologic signs

    1. Bilateral ptosis

    2. Progressive external ophthalmoplegia

    3. Myotonia of lid closure and gaze holding

    4. Orbicularis weaknesses

 5. Polychromatophilic cataracts
 6. Miotic pupils, sluggish to light and near
 7. Retinal pigmentary degeneration

D. Multiple systemic findings include face, neck, and limb myopathy with atrophy, testicular atrophy, baldness, cardiac conduction defects

V. **Dysthyroid myopathy (Graves' disease)**

A. A restrictive myopathy occurring commonly in middle-aged and elderly individuals, leading to ophthalmoparesis and diplopia

B. Lymphocytic and plasmacytic infiltration of extraocular muscles; leads to edema, activation of fibroblasts with production of acid mucopolysaccharide and fibrosis

C. Variety of ocular motility patterns produced
 1. "Elevator palsy" due to fibrotic shortening of the inferior rectus
 2. "Abduction weaknesses" due to involvement of the medial rectus, mimicking a VI nerve palsy
 3. Superior and lateral rectus muscles less frequently involved
 4. Frequency of clinical involvement of rectus muscles: IR > MR > SR > LR

D. Additional findings include:
 1. Proptosis
 2. Lids: retraction, lid lag on downward gaze (von Graefe's sign), edema
 3. Conjunctiva: injection over horizontal rectus muscles, chemosis
 4. Cornea: keratopathy, erosions, ulceration
 5. Optic neuropathy due to compression at orbital apex by enlarged extraocular muscles (see Chapter 9)

E. Table 11-1 summarizes clinical findings with "NO SPECS" mnemonic classification and soft-tissue involvement with "RELIEF" mnemonic

F. Diagnostic studies
 1. Forced duction testing (see Chapter 20)
 2. Ultrasonography to measure size of extraocular muscles
 3. Orbital computed tomography (CT) scanning
  a. Typically enlargement of all extraocular muscles in both orbits
  b. Muscle tendon spared
 4. Thyroid function tests

G. Association of dysthyroidism with myasthenia; two diseases may coexist and give a variety of ocular findings

VI. **Idiopathic orbital inflammation (orbital pseudotumor)**

A. A syndrome occurring in any age group consisting of acute onset of orbital pain, chemosis, conjunctival injection, and frequently proptosis

B. If the inflammatory process affects one or more of the extraocular muscles, the term orbital myositis is employed. These patients typically complain of diplopia

C. Pathologic studies in such cases demonstrate orbital structures (blood vessels, muscles, lacrimal glands, etc) infiltrated with chronic inflammatory cells

D. In the vast majority of cases, the etiology of the inflammatory response is unknown,

Table 11-1

GRAVES' DISEASE SIGNS (MNEMONIC)

N o signs or symptoms

O nly signs of lid retraction, lid lag, stare

S oft tissue signs and symptoms:

> **R** esistance to retropulsion
>
> **E** dema of conjunctiva and caruncle
>
> **L** acrimal gland enlargement
>
> **I** njection over rectus muscle insertion
>
> **E** dema of eyelids
>
> **F** ullness of eyelids

P roptosis

E xtraocular muscle enlargement

C orneal exposure secondary to exposure

S ight loss secondary to optic nerve compression

Modified from Van Dyk HJ. Orbital Graves' disease. A modification of the NO SPECS classification. *Ophthalmology.* 1981;88:479-483.

---

 although it may occur with systemic disorders, including lupus erythematosus, rheumatoid arthritis, sarcoidosis, Wegener's granulomatosis, dermatomyositis

E. Diagnostic studies

 1. Orbital ultrasonography

 2. Orbital CT scanning

  a. Usually only one or two extraocular muscles enlarged in a single orbit (myositis)

  b. Muscle tendon enlarged as well

 3. Orbital biopsy

F. Treatment modalities

 1. Systemic steroids usually produce dramatic improvement in symptoms in 24 to 48 hours with clearing of signs over 1 to 4 weeks

 2. Orbital radiation therapy: 1000 to 2000 cGy

 3. Chlorambucil or cyclophosphamide for chronic, recurrent orbital pseudotumor

G. It may be difficult to distinguish between benign orbital inflammation and orbital lymphoma, both clinically and pathologically. All patients with idiopathic orbital inflammation must be followed carefully. An initial salutary response to steroid therapy by no means excludes a malignant process

Bibliography

Books

Char DH. *Thyroid Eye Disease.* 3rd ed. New York, NY: Butterworth-Heinemann; 1997.

Gorman CA, Waller RR, Dyer JA. *The Eye and Orbit in Thyroid Disease.* New York, NY: Raven Press; 1984.

Lisak RP, Barchi RL. *Myasthenia Gravis and Myasthenic Syndromes.* New York, NY: Marcel Dekker; 1994.

Rootman J. *Diseases of the Orbit.* Philadelphia, Pa: JB Lippincott; 1988.

Chapters

Glaser JS, Siatkowski RM. Infranuclear disorders of eye movement. In: Duane TD, ed. *Clinical Ophthalmology.* Vol 2. Philadelphia, Pa: Lippincott-Williams & Wilkins; 1998: 35-63.

Karsh JW, Baer JC, Henady RK. Noninfectious orbital inflammatory disease. In: Duane TD, ed. *Clinical Ophthalmology.* Philadelphia, Pa: Lippincott-Williams & Wilkins; 1994: 1-45.

Kuncl RW, Hoffman PN. Myopathies and disorders of neuromuscular transmission. In: Miller NR, Newman NJ, eds. *Clinical Neuro-ophthalmology.* Vol 1. 5th ed. Baltimore, Md: Williams & Wilkins; 1998: 1351-1460.

Skalka HW. Ultrasonography in the diagnosis of endocrine orbitopathy. In: Smith JL, ed. *Neuro-Ophthalmology Focus 1980.* New York, NY: Masson; 1979: 211-216.

Articles

Cogan DG. Myasthenia gravis: a review of the disease and a description of lid twitch as a characteristic sign. *Arch Ophthalmol.* 1965;74:217-221.

Drachman DA. Ophthalmoplegia plus: the neuro-degenerative disorders associated with progressive external Ophthalmoplegia. *Arch Neurol.* 1968;18:654-674.

Drachman DB. Myasthenia gravis. *N Engl J Med.* 1994;330:1747-1810.

Dresner SC, Kennerdell JS. Dysthyroid orbitopathy. *Neurology.* 1985;35:1628-1634.

Garrity JA, Fatourechi V, Bergstralh EJ, et al. Results of orbital decompression in 428 patients with severe Graves' ophthalmopathy. *Am J Ophthalmol.* 1993;116:533-547.

Glaser JS. Myasthenic pseudo-internuclear ophthalmoplegia. *Arch Ophthalmol.* 1966;75:363-366.

Gorelick PB, Pena R, Lee AG et al. An ice test for the diagnosis of myasthenia gravis. *Ophthalmology.* 1999;106:1282-1286.

Kearns TB, Sayre GP. Retinitis pigmentosa, external ophthalmoplegia and complete heart block. *Arch Ophthalmol.* 1958;60:280-289.

Kennerdell JS. Management of nonspecific inflammatory and lymphoid orbital lesions. *Int Ophthalmol Clin.* 1991;31:7-15.

Kennerdell JS, Dresner SC. The nonspecific orbital inflammatory syndromes. *Surv Ophthalmol.* 1984;29:92-113.

Lloyd WC, Leone CR. Supervoltage orbital radiotherapy in 36 cases of Graves' disease. *Am J Ophthalmol.* 1992;113:374-380.

Moorhty G, Behrens MB, Drachman DB, et al. Ocular pseudomyasthenia or ocular myasthenia "plus." *Neurology.* 1989;39:1150-1154.

Newman NJ. Mitochondrial diseases and the eye. *Ophthamol Clin NA.* 1992;5:405-424.

Odel JG, Winterkorn JMS, Behrens MM. The sleep test for myasthenia gravis. *J Clin Neuro-ophthalmol.* 1991;11:288-292.

Osserman KE, Kaplan LI. Rapid diagnostic test for myasthenia gravis: increased muscle strength, without fasciculations, after intravenous administration of edrophonium (Tensilon) chloride. *JAMA.* 1952;150:265-269.

Rootman J, Nugent R. The classification and management of acute orbital pseudotumors. *Ophthalmology.* 1982;89:1040-1048.

Spoor TC, Martinez AJ, Kennerdell JS, et al. Dysthyroid and myasthenia myopathy of the medial rectus: a clinical pathologic report. *Neurology.* 1980;30:939-944.

Steele JC, Richardson JC, Olsewski J. Progressive supranuclear palsy. *Arch Neurol.* 1964;10:333-359.

Van Dyk HJ. Orbital Graves' disease. A modification of the NO SPECS classification. *Ophthalmology.* 1981;88:479-483.

Chapter 12

V Nerve (Trigeminal) Syndromes

I. **Anatomical considerations (Figure 12-1)**

A. The trigeminal nerve is a mixed nerve:

1. Sensory—ipsilateral side of face

2. Motor—ipsilateral muscles of mastication (masseter, temporalis, pterygoids)

B. Nuclear complex

1. Sensory portion of trigeminal nerve extends from the midbrain to the upper cervical cord

2. Mesencephalic (rostral) nucleus—proprioception and deep sensation from tendons and muscles of mastication

3. Main sensory nucleus

   a. Located in pons

   b. Subserves light touch

4. Spinal nucleus

   a. Extends from pons to upper cervical cord

   b. Subserves pain and temperature

   c. Divided into segments that correspond to dermatomes that are concentric around the mouth

C. Peripheral nerve

1. The trigeminal nerve supplies sensation to the ipsilateral side of the face via three branches

   a. V^1—Ophthalmic division: frontal, lacrimal, and nasociliary

   b. V^2—Maxillary division: cheek and lower eyelid

   c. V^3—Mandibular division: area of mandible (but not angle of mandible), lower lip, tongue

2. Motor nucleus lies in pons medially to main sensory nucleus and axons travel with mandibular (V^3) division

3. Three divisions of trigeminal nerve converge at trigeminal (Gasserian) ganglion, which lies in Meckel's cave of temporal bone

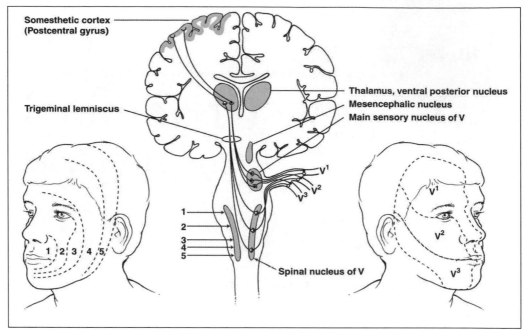

Figure 12-1. Diagram of the central pathways and peripheral innervation of the V nerve.

       4. Fibers then travel through main sensory root to brainstem

II. Oculofacial hypesthesia (see Figure 12-1)

  A. Distribution of facial numbness or paresthesias helps determine central or peripheral origin

      1. Concentric perioral numbness/parestheisa—central (nuclear) origin (eg, ischemia, demyelination)

      2. Band of numbness/paresthesia—peripheral origin (ie, V^1, V^2, V^3)

      3. Such somatotopic hypesthesia (eg, V^2 only, or V^2 and V^3 with sparing of V^1) suggests that the lesion is more likely to be in the middle cranial fossa (cavernous sinus) or orbit

  B. Differential diagnosis of diminished sensation in the trigeminal distribution[*]

      1. Corneal

         a. Herpes simplex

         b. Herpes zoster

         c. Ocular surgery

         d. Cerebellopontine angle tumors

         e. Dysautonomia

         f. Congenital

      2. Ophthalmic division

         a. Neoplasm, orbital apex

         b. Neoplasm, superior orbital fissure

---

*From Glaser JS. Neuro-ophthalmology. In: Duane TD, ed. *Clinical Ophthalmology*. Vol 2. Philadelphia, Pa: Lippincott-Williams & Wilkins; 1994: chapter 3, 17-19.

      c. Neoplasm, cavernous sinus

      d. Neoplasm, middle fossa

      e. Aneurysm, cavernous sinus

  3. Maxillary division

      a. Orbit floor fracture

      b. Maxillary antrum carcinoma

      c. Perineural spread of skin carcinoma

      d. Neoplasm, foremen rotundum, sphenopterygoid fossa

  4. Mandibular division

      a. Nasopharyngeal tumor

      b. Middle fossa tumor

  5. All divisions

      a. Nasopharyngeal carcinoma

      b. Cerebellopontine angle tumors

      c. Brainstem lesions (dissociated sensory loss)

      d. Intracavernous aneurysm

      e. Demyelinative

      f. Middle fossa or Meckel's cave tumor

      g. Benign sensory neuropathy

      h. Tentorial meningioma

      i. Toxins (eg, trichlorethylene)

      j. Trigeminal neurofibroma

III. Oculofacial pain

A. Differential diagnosis of relatively common entities associated with ocular and facial pain*

  1. Ocular

      a. Local corneal, lid, and anterior segment disease

      b. Ocular inflammation

      c. Dry eye and tear deficiency syndromes

      d. Chronic ocular hypoxia, carotid occlusive disease

  2. Ophthalmic division

      a. Migraine, cluster headaches

      b. Raeder's paratrigeminal neuralgia

      c. Painful ophthalmoplegia syndromes

      d. Herpes zoster—nasociliary nerve involvement indicated by vesicular eruption on side or tip of nose (Hutchison's sign)

      e. Referred (dural) pain, including occipital infarction

      f. Tic douloureux (infrequent in V^1)

      g. Sinusitis

  3. Maxillary division

      a. Tic douloureux

      b. Nasopharyngeal carcinoma

      c. Tempomandibular syndrome

      d. Dental disease

      e. Sinusitis

      4. Mandibular division
         a. Tic douloureux
         b. Dental disease
      5. Miscellaneous
         a. Atypical facial neuralgias
         b. Pain with medullary lesions (eg, Wallenberg syndrome)
         c. Giant cell arteritis (see Chapter 9)
         d. Trigeminal tumors

B. Specific trigeminal syndromes
    1. Referred pain
        a. Any intracranial process irritating the dural sensory fibers, which may be supplied by recurrent branches of V nerve
        b. Neck pain (eg, from osteoarthritis in the cervical spine) may be referred to the eye because of the cervical sensory fibers traveling with the trigeminal fibers of the spinal tract of V, which extends to C-2 level
    2. Trigeminal neuralgia (tic douloureux)
        a. Paroxysmal pain in the distribution of one or more of the divisions of V (V^3 > V^2 > V^1)
        b. Recurring, lancinating, "lightning" hemifacial pain lasting 20 to 30 seconds
        c. Pain may be so intense that the facial muscles contract and distort the face during an attack. Frequently "triggered" by touching certain areas of the face or scalp; asymptomatic or mild headache between episodes
        d. No neurologic deficits (including normal corneal reflex)
        e. Neuralgia of more persistent nature and associated with neurologic deficits may resolve from compressive, demylinative, or inflammatory lesion of the V nerve
    3. Herpetic neuralgia
        a. Pain of herpes zoster is described as severe, burning, aching in quality
        b. Pain occurs over distribution of a dermatome or cranial nerve, usually V^1, although it may involve the facial nerve (external ear) with ipsilateral facial palsy (Ramsay-Hunt syndrome)
        c. Pain often precedes onset of typical rash by 4 to 7 days
        d. Pain usually regresses within 1 to 2 weeks, but may persist for months or years: post-herpetic neuralgia
        e. Patients typically describe dysesthesias as "crawling" and "prickly" sensations
    4. Raeder's paratrigeminal neuralgia
        a. V nerve distribution pain with ipsilateral Horner's syndrome
        b. Almost exclusively in middle-aged or elderly male patients
        c. May be caused by migrainous dilation of the internal carotid artery with compression of the V nerve and sympathetic plexus in the middle cranial fossa
        d. If the pain is persistent (not of migrainous episodic nature) or if associated with cranial nerve palsy, then suspect a middle fossa tumor, aneurysm, or internal carotid artery dissection

BIBLIOGRAPHY

Books

Fromm GH, Sessle BJ. *Trigeminal Neuralgia: Current Concepts Regarding Pathogenesis and Treatment.* Boston, Mass: Butterworth-Heinemann; 1991.

Chapters

Glaser JS. Neuro-ophthalmology. In: Duane TD, ed. *Clinical Ophthalmology.* Vol 2. Philadelphia, Pa: Lippincott-Williams & Wilkins; 1998: chapter 3, 15-19.

Lavin PJM. Ocular and facial pain syndromes. In: Rosen ES, Eustace P, Thompson HS, Cumming WJK, eds. *Neuro-ophthalmology.* St. Louis, Mo: Mosby; 1998: chapter 23, 1-18.

Martin TJ, Corbett JJ. *Neuro-ophthalmology—The Requisites.* St. Louis, Mo: Mosby; 2000: 223-232.

Miller NR, Newman NJ, eds. *Walsh and Hoyt's Clinical Neuro-ophthalmology.* 5th ed. Vol 1. Baltimore, Md: Williams & Wilkins; 1998: chapters 33-35.

Articles

Aviel A, Marshak G. Ramsay-Hunt syndrome: a cranial polyneuropathy. *Am J Otolaryngol.* 1982;3:61-66.

Davis RH, Daroff RB, Hoyt WF. Hemicrania, oculosympathetic paresis, and subcranial carotid aneurysm: Raeder's paratrigeminal syndrome (Group 2). *J Neurosurg.* 1968;29:94-96.

Feindel W, Penfield W, McNaughton F. The tentorial nerves and localization of intracranial pain in man. *Neurology.* 1960;10:555-563.

Grimson BS, Thompson HS. Raeder's syndrome: a clinical review. *Surv Ophthalmol.* 1980;25:199-210.

Kline LB, Vitek JJ, Raymon BC. Painful Horner's syndrome due to spontaneous carotid artery dissection. *Ophthalmology.* 1987;94:226-230.

Kust RG, Straus SE. Postherpetic neuralgia: pathogenesis, treatment and prevention. *N Engl J Med.* 1996;335:32-42.

Smith JL. Raeder's paratrigeminal syndrome. *Am J Ophthalmol.* 1958;46:194-201.

Trobe JD, Hood CL, Parsons JT, et al. Intracranial spread of squamous carcinoma along the trigeminal nerve. *Arch Ophthalmol.* 1982;100:608-611.

Chapter 13

The Seven Syndromes of the VII Nerve (Facial)

I. **Anatomical considerations**

A. Figure 13-1 is a schematic representation of the course of the supranuclear and infranuclear fibers controlling the facial musculature. The fibers are accompanied by the nervus intermedius (tearing, salivation, taste), as well as sensory fibers from the external ear and the nerve to the stapedius muscle. The nerve leaves the pons and travels with the VIII cranial nerve through the internal auditory canal, leaving the canal through the fallopian canal, which courses inferiorly through the petrous bone, exiting through the stylomastoid foramen

II. **The seven syndromes of the VII nerve**

A. Supranuclear facial palsy (see Figure 13-1, site 1) results in contralateral weakness of the lower two-thirds of the face, with some weakness of the orbicularis oculi, but not as severe as with peripheral VII nerve palsy (Figures 13-2a and 13-2b); does not usually require tarsorrhaphy

B. Cerebellopontine angle tumor (see Figure 13-1, site 2)
   1. Total ipsilateral facial weakness
   2. Decreased tearing (nervus intermedius)
   3. Hyperacusis (nerve to stapedius muscle)
   4. Decreased taste of anterior two-thirds of tongue (nervus intermedius and chorda tympani)
   5. Associated neurologic deficits: V, VI, VIII, Horner's syndrome, gaze palsy, nystagmus (see Chapter 3, Section X), papilledema, cerebellar dysfunction

C. Geniculate ganglionitis (Ramsay-Hunt syndrome, zoster oticus [see Figure 13-1, site 3])
   1. Same findings as Figure 13-1, site 2; no associated neurologic deficits except for possibly a VIII nerve involvement (hearing loss, vestibular dysfunction)
   2. May see zoster vesicles in areas supplied by sensory portion of VII nerve: tympanic membrane, external auditory canal, pinna, buccal mucosa, neck
   3. Recovery is poorer than with Bell's palsy (see below)

D. Isolated ipsilateral tear deficiency (see Figure 13-1, site 4)

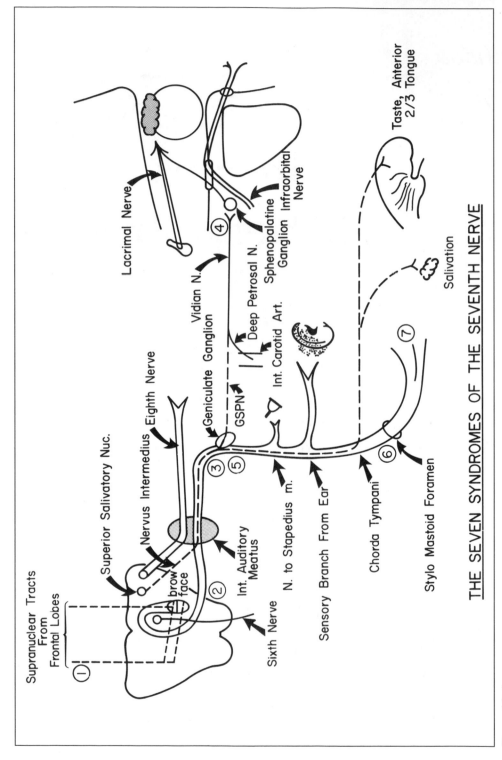

THE SEVEN SYNDROMES OF THE SEVENTH NERVE

Figure 13-1.

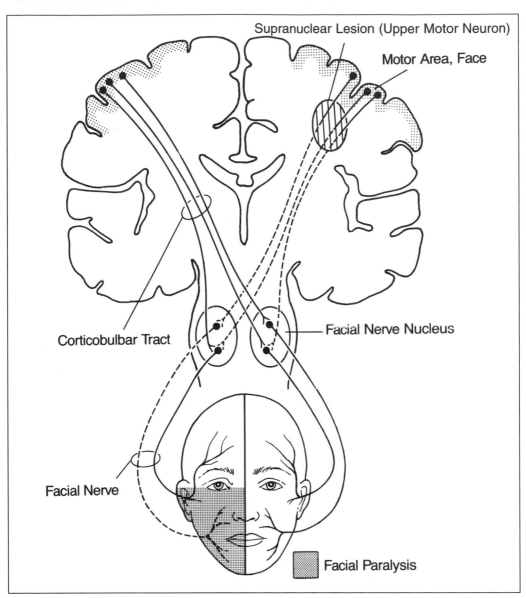

Figure 13-2a. Facial weakness due to an upper motor neuron lesion.

    1. Nasopharyngeal carcinoma may affect the vidian nerve or sphenopalatine ganglion; often accompanying VI nerve palsy due to cavernous sinus involvement

E. Bell's palsy (see Figure 13-1, site 5)

    1. Common idiopathic facial palsy, possibly due to viral infection and edema of VII nerve within fallopian canal

    2. Same findings as Figure 13-1, site 2 except for no associated neurologic deficits; tearing may be normal

    3. Complete recovery, within 60 days in 75% of patients; with steroid therapy, recovery over 90%

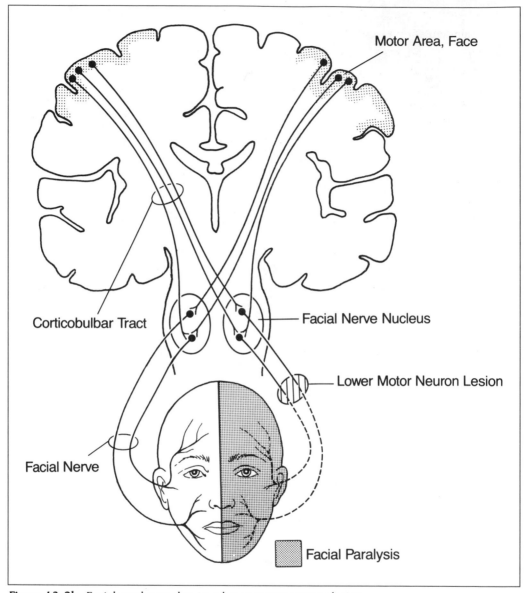

Figure 13-2b. Facial weakness due to a lower motor neuron lesion.

      4. Antiviral agents often used: acyclovir, famciclovir

  F. Isolated total ipsilateral facial palsy (see Figure 13-1, site 6)

      1. Mastoidopathy, facial trauma, parotid gland surgery

  G. Isolated partial ipsilateral facial palsy (see Figure 13-1, site 7)

      1. Only certain branches of VII nerve are affected

III. Facial diplegia

  A. Brainstem contusion

B. Brainstem stroke (basilar artery)

C. Brainstem glioma

D. Moebius syndrome: aplasia of VII nerve nuclei in brainstem; often accompanied by:
   1. Bilateral VI nerve palsies
   2. Palatal and lingual palsy
   3. Deafness
   4. Deficiencies of pectoral and lingual muscles
   5. Extremity defects: syndactyly, supernumary digits, absent fingers and toes

E. Myasthenia gravis (see Chapter 11)

F. Guillain-Barré syndrome (see Chapter 7, Section V, G)

G. Myotonic dystrophy (see Chapter 11, Section IV)

H. Melkersson-Rosenthal syndrome
   1. Rare, idiopathic disorder
   2. Facial swelling
   3. Transversely fissured tongue
   4. Recurrent, alternating facial palsy

I. Neoplastic: leukemia, meningeal carcinomatosis

J. Inflammatory: sarcoidosis, porphyria

K. Infectious: polio, AIDS, Lyme disease

IV. Crocodile tears (gustolacrimal reflex)

A. Any patient with VII nerve palsy that has affected the parasympathetic fibers stimulating tearing and salivation may experience tearing at mealtime due to aberrant regeneration or misdirection of fibers, so that when neural stimulus for salivation is transmitted, it results in stimulation of tearing

V. Spastic paretic facial contracture

A. Unilateral spastic facial contracture with associated facial weakness

B. Indicative of intrinsic pontine neoplasm

C. Due to damage of VII nerve nucleus (facial paresis) and its supranuclear connections (facial spasticity)

VI. Blepharospasm

A. Onset usually in adult life (sixth and seventh decade); 3:1 female predominance

B. Bilateral, episodic, involuntary contractions of the orbicularis oculi

C. At times, associated with involuntary spasm of the lower facial musculature: orofacial dyskinesia or Meige's syndrome

D. Etiology
   1. Adults
      a. Usually unknown ("essential" blepharospasm); possibly related to dysfunction of the basal ganglia and limbic system
      b. May occur in patients with Parkinson's disease, progressive supranuclear palsy, Huntington's disease, multiple sclerosis, and brainstem stroke

    2. Children

      a. Usually benign, self-limited habit

      b. Tourette's syndrome

  E. Treatment

    1. Pharmacologic: clonazepam (Klonopin)

    2. Chemodenervation: botulinum toxin

    3. Surgery: selective VII nerve sectioning; orbicularis myectomies

VII. Hemifacial spasm

A. Unilateral (rarely bilateral) spasm involving half of facial muscles, typically lasting several minutes at a time; persists during sleep

B. Painless, no sensory loss

C. Etiology

    1. Aberrant vascular loop (dolichoectasia) compressing VII nerve in subarachnoid space where it exits the pons

    2. Following Bell's palsy (postparalytic hemifacial spasm)

D. Treatment

    1. Pharmachologic: carbamazepine, baclofen, clonazepam, neurontin

    2 Chemodenervation: botulinum toxin

    3 Surgery: posterior fossa craniotomy with insertion of inert material between vascular loop and VII nerve

VIII. Facial myokymia

A. Usually benign, self-limited

B. If persistent over weeks or months, then consider:

    1. Multiple sclerosis

    2. Brainstem glioma

    3. Brainstem stroke

BIBLIOGRAPHY

Books

Jankovic J, Hallett M, eds. *Therapy with Botulinum Toxin.* New York, NY: Marcel Dekker; 1994.

Chapters

Burde RM, Savino PJ, Trobe JD. *Clinical Decisions in Neuro-ophthalmology.* St. Louis, Mo: Mosby-Year Book; 1992: 347-378.

Galetta S, May M. The facial nerve and related disorders of the face. In: Duane TD, ed. *Clinical Ophthalmology.* Philadelphia, Pa: Lippincott-Williams & Wilkins; 1998: chapter 8, 1-39.

Articles

Austin JR, Peskind SP, Austin SG, et al. Idiopathic facial nerve paralysis: a randomized double-blind controlled study of placebo versus prednisone. *Laryngoscope.* 1993;103:1326-1333.

Bauer CA, Coker NJ. Update on facial nerve disorders. *Otolaryngol Clin NA.* 1996;29:445-454.

Elston JS. The management of blepharospasm and hemifacial spasm. *J Neurol.* 1992;239:5-8.

Frueh DR, Felt DP, Wojno JH, et al. Treatment of blepharospasm with botulinum toxin. *Arch Ophthalmol.* 1984;102:1146-1468.

Gillum WN, Anderson RL. Blepharospasm surgery: an anatomical approach. *Arch Ophthalmol.* 1981;99:1056-1062.

Jankovic J, Havins WE, Wilkins RB. Blinking and blepharospasm: mechanics, diagnosis and management. *JAMA.* 1982;248:3160-3164.

Jannetta PJ. The cause of hemifacial spasm: definitive microsurgical treatment at the brainstem in 31 patients. *Trans Am Acad Ophthalmol Otolaryngol.* 1974;80:319-322.

Sogg RL, Hoyt WF, Boldrey E. Spastic paretic facial contraction: a rare sign of brainstem tumor. *Neurology.* 1963;13:607-612.

Chapter 14

Eyelid Disorders

Saunders L. Hupp, MD

I. **Anatomical considerations (Figure 14-1)**

  A. Eyelid opening and closing is mediated through three muscle groups

    1. Levator palpebrae: elevator of upper eyelid

    2. Muller's muscles of eyelids: in lower lid, also known as inferior tarsal muscle

    3. Orbicularis oculi: closure of upper and lower lids

  B. Innervation of three muscle groups

    1. Levator palpebrae: superior division of III nerve (see Figure 5-1)

    2. Muller's muscles of eyelids: third-order neuron of oculosympathetic pathway (see Figure 8-3)

    3. Orbicularis oculi: VII nerve (see Figure 13-2)

II. **Physiology of eyelid opening**

  A. Supranuclear control of eyelid opening is through both corticobulbar and extrapyramidal pathways. Areas of the frontal, occipital, and temporal cortex have been associated with eyelid opening. Also, the arousal state of the brain influences palpebral fissure width through control of levator tonus

  B. Final common pathway for eyelid opening:

    1. Central caudal subnucleus of III nerve nuclear complex to both levator palpebrae muscles

    2. Fibers to the levator muscle travel with the superior division of III nerve

  C. Physiologic synkineses link the activity of the levator muscles to related extraocular and facial muscle movement

    1. Movements of the upper eyelids are identically coordinated, obeying Herring's law of equal innervation. The eyelids lift with upgaze and lower with downgaze

    2. Inverse relationship between superior recess and eyelid movement during sleep and with forced eyelid closure. Bell's phenomenon: globe movement up and out as lids close

    3. Voluntary reflex blinking: inhibition of levator tonus occurs with stimulation of the VII nerve, indicating interconnections between the central caudal nucleus of III nerve and VII nerve nucleus

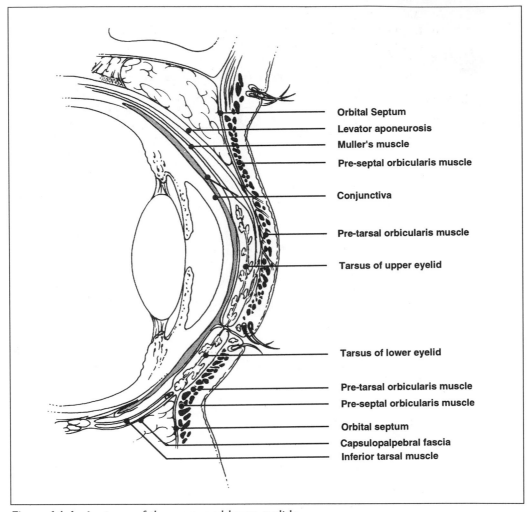

Orbital Septum
Levator aponeurosis
Muller's muscle
Pre-septal orbicularis muscle

Conjunctiva

Pre-tarsal orbicularis muscle

Tarsus of upper eyelid

Tarsus of lower eyelid

Pre-tarsal orbicularis muscle
Pre-septal orbicularis muscle

Orbital septum
Capsulopalpebral fascia
Inferior tarsal muscle

Figure 14-1. Anatomy of the upper and lower eyelids.

III.   Abnormalities of eyelid opening

A. Ptosis—insufficient opening of the eyelid; may be congenital or acquired

1. Congenital ptosis—may be unilateral or bilateral, and may be associated with other congenital ocular or orbital abnormalities

    a. Marcus Gunn jaw winking phenomenon

        i.   Most common synkinetic movement associated with congenital ptosis

        ii. External pterygoid—levator synkinesis: elevation of lid with movement of mandible to opposite side, protruded forward, or wide opening of the mouth

        iii. Internal pterygoid—levator synkinesis: elevation of the lid with clenching of the teeth

    b. Blepharophimosis syndrome—triad: bilateral ptosis, telecanthus, phimosis of lid fissures

c. Anophthalmos (absence of eye)

d. Eyelid hamartomas (eg, S-shaped lid from neurofibromatosis)

e. Co-existent strabismus or amblyopia

f. Congenital fibrosis of the extraocular muscles

g. Superior rectus weakness (double elevator palsy)

2. Acquired ptosis

   a. Neurogenic

      i. Unilateral temporal, occipital or bilateral frontal cortical lesions may produce unilateral or bilateral "cortical ptosis" via interruption of supranuclear pathways

         a. Apraxia of eyelid opening: unusual form of ptosis occasionally associated with extrapyramidal disease, such as Parkinson's disease, or progressive supranuclear palsy

         b. Supranuclear ptosis may appear in patients with hysterical or functional disease

      ii. Paradoxic supranuclear inhibition of levator tonus

         a. Resultant ptosis may be isolated or associated with congenital horizontal or vertical eye movement abnormalities

         b. Inverse Marcus Gunn phenomenon:

            i. Eyelid closure during mouth opening

            ii. With downward movement of lower jaw, there is total inhibition of levator with subsequent ptosis

      iii. Lesions of the III nerve (Chapter 5)

      iv. Lesions of the oculosympathetic pathway

      v. Ophthalmoplegic migraine (Chapter 15)

      vi. Horner's syndrome (Chapter 8)

         a. Ptosis is mild, usually less than 3 mm

         b. "Upside-down" ptosis: relaxation of the inferior tarsal muscle

   b. Myogenic

      i. Myasthenia gravis (Chapter 11)

         a. Initial manifestation in up to 75% of patients

         b. Variable, typically worsens with fatigue

         c. May be produced by having patient sustain upgaze

         d. Look for Cogan's lid twitch sign (Chapter 11)

         e. Frequently associated with orbicularis weakness

         f. May be accompanied by ocular motility disturbances

         g. On occasion, may have coexistent eye signs of thyroid eye disease

         h. With asymmetric ptosis, patient uses frontalis muscle to elevate both lids—produces lid retraction on one side, with manual elevation of more ptotic lid, the previously retracted lid falls—phenomenon termed "enhanced ptosis" (due to Herring's law of equal innervation to both levator muscles)

         i. **Remember:** Consider Tensilon testing in all patients with onset of acquired isolated ptosis

      ii. Chronic progressive external ophthalmoplegia (Chapter 11)

   iii. Myotonic dystrophy (Chapter 11)

   iv. Botulism (Chapter 7)

   v. Corticosteroid-induced ptosis

    a. Long-term topical corticosteroid therapy (eg, uveitis)

    b. May be a localized form of steroid myopathy

  c. Aponeurotic

   i. Typical features

    a. Ptosis consistent in all positions of gaze

    b. Good levator function (>10 mm)

    c. Raised skin crease

    d. Deep upper lid sulcus

    e. Thinned upper lid may be almost transparent

   ii. May have associated bulging fat if defect extends to musculo-aponeu-rotic junction

   iii. Most common cause of "senile" or "involutional" ptosis

   iv. At surgery, find dchiscence in levator aponeurosis and/or disinsertion of aponeurosis from tarsal plate of upper lid

  d. Traumatic

   i. Lid laceration

   ii. Postsurgical (eg, following cataract surgery, orbital surgery)

   iii. Intraorbital foreign body

   iv. Orbital roof fracture

  e. Mechanical

   i. Eyelid tumor

   ii. Eyelid infiltration (eg, amyloidosis, lymphoma)

   iii. Brow or upper facial laxity and droop

   iv. Contact lens wear

   v. Blepharochalasis

   vi. Cicatricial—damage following surgery, chemical or thermal injury, or inflammation (trachoma, ocular pemphigoid)

  f. Pseudoptosis—look for abnormalities of facial, orbital, or ocular anatomy

   i. Microphthalmia

   ii. Phthisis bulbi

   iii. Enophthalmos

   iv. Dermatochalasis

   v. Hypotropia

   vi. Contralateral lid retraction

B. Lid retraction or excessive elevation—characterized by sclera visible above superior corneal limbus when the eyes are directed straight ahead

 1. Neuropathic lid retraction

  a. Supranuclear retraction

   i. Often associated with lesions of the rostral dorsal midbrain in the region of the posterior commissure (Collier's sign)

   ii. Combination of lid retraction with downward displacement of eyes in infants produces the "setting sun" sign

      iii. Periodic lid retraction may occur as isolated myoclonic movement or as part of vertical nystagmus seen with ocular myoclonus (see Chapter 3)

      iv. Comatose patient may demonstrate periodic lid retraction synchronous with breathing or head movements

  b. Lid retraction from paradoxic levator excitation may be congenital or acquired

    i. Congenital lid retraction may be seen with abnormalities of horizontal gaze (Duane's syndrome), jaw movements (Marcus Gunn phenomenon), or swallowing

    ii. Acquired eyelid retraction associated with aberrant regeneration following III nerve palsy (pseudo von Graefe's sign)

    iii. Claude Bernard syndrome: irritative lesion of oculosympathetic pathway produces lid retraction and an enlarged ipsilateral pupil (opposite of Horner's syndrome)

    iv. Lid retraction may be physiologic response (Herring's law) to ptosis of the contralateral eye

2. Neuromuscular eyelid retraction

  a. Patients with myasthenia gravis without evidence of thyroid disease

  b. Sympathomimetic drops (phenylephrine) stimulate Muller's muscles of eyelids

3. Myopathic lid retraction

  a. Most common form of lid retraction due to thyroid eye disease. Congenital transient lid retraction may be associated with maternal hyperthyroidism

  b. Maldevelopment of the levator muscle

  c. Hepatic cirrhosis

4. Eyelid lag—lack of inhibition of upper eyelids on downgaze

  a. Most commonly associated with lid retraction due to thyroid eye disease

  b. Lid lag without lid retraction may occur in extrapyramidal syndromes with lesions of the midbrain involving the nucleus of the posterior commissure

    i. Parkinson's disease

    ii. Progressive supranuclear palsy

    iii. Thalamic-midbrain infarction

IV. Physiology of eyelid closure

A. Lid closure may be:

  1. Bilateral: blink

  2. Unilateral: wink

B. Cortical control of lid closure via bilateral corticobulbar pathways with predominant innervation to contralateral side

C. Subcortical control mediated through extrapyramidal pathways that are affected by emotional states and tension

D. Extrapyramidal control may be absent in infants or synchronized with mouth movements, such as sucking

E. Peripheral pathway to orbicularis oculi via VII nerve (see Figure 13-1)

F. With each blink, there is complete inhibition of the levator just prior (10 milliseconds) to onset of contraction of orbicularis oculi

---

Table 14-1

PHYSIOLOGIC SYNKINESES AND REFLEX BLINKING

Reflex	Clinical examination
Orbicularis stress	Tap lateral orbicularis oculi
Corneal blink	Corneal touch (V^1 nerve)
Cochleopalpebral	Sudden noise
Auropalpebral	Stimulate external auditory canal
Palatal palpebral	Touch palate
Bright flash	Rapid exposure to bright light

G. Normal or periodic blink
   1. 12 to 16 per minute in relaxed state
   2. Decreased with reading or concentration
   3. Increased with emotion (anxiety or arousal)
   4. Protects and nourishes avascular cornea
   5. Facilitates eye movement (saccade) to change direction of gaze

H. Reflex control of blinking is mediated though a variety of physiologic synkineses (Table 14-1)

V.   **Abnormalities of eyelid closure**

A. Insufficiency of eyelid closure
   1. Supranuclear facial palsy
   2. VII nerve palsy
   3. Myasthenia gravis—"peek" phenomenon: after sustained lid closure of orbicularis oculi, lid opening occurs due to orbicularis fatigue
   4. Systemic disease
      a. Muscular dystrophy
      b. Myotonic dystrophy
      c. Chronic progressive external ophthalmoplegia
   5. After surgery involving recession of the inferior rectus muscle

B. Decreased blink rate
   1. Parkinson's disease
   2. Thyroid eye disease
   3. Progressive supranuclear palsy
   4. Infants in first few months of life

C. Excessive eyelid closure—pathologic blinking or blepharospasm
   1. Supranuclear cause of blepharospasm
      a. Focal seizure
      b. Reflex blepharospasm (post-stroke)
      c. Response to ocular irritation
      d. Associated with tardive dyskinesia

       e. Post-encephalitis

       f. Hysterical

       g. Habit spasms and tics (eg, Tourette's syndrome)

       h. Orofacial dyskinesia—Meige's syndrome

       i. Essential blepharospasm

2. Brainstem disease associated with decreased eye movements may require a blink to facilitate a saccade through a blink-saccade synkinesis

       a. Huntington's chorea

       b. Gaucher's disease

       c. Parkinson's disease

       d. Congenital ocular motor apraxia

3. Primary brainstem disease

       a. Brainstem stroke

       b. Demyelinating disease

       c. Trauma

4. Benign facial or eyelid myokymia

5. Spastic paretic facial contracture (see Chapter 13)

       a. Facial myokymia with contracture plus weakness of facial muscles

       b. Etiologies:

           i. Intra-axial (pons): tumor, stroke, multiple sclerosis

           ii. Extra-axial: cerebellopontine angle mass, Bell's palsy, Guillain-Barré syndrome

6. Peripheral facial nerve disease (see Chapter 13)

       a. Hemifacial spasm—"idiopathic": high percentage of cases may be due to dolichoectasia of vertebral and/or basilar arteries with compression of dorsal root entry zone of VII nerve

       b. Postparalytic hemifacial spasm (following facial palsy)

7. Neuromuscular disease

       a. Tetany

       b. Strychnine poisoning

       c. Tetanus (risus sardonicus)

8. Systemic disease

       a. Hypothyroidism

       b. Myotonic dystrophy

       c. Hyperkalemic familial paralysis

       d. Chondrodystrophic dystonia (Schwartz-Jampel syndrome)

D. Eyelid nystagmus

1. Rhythmic oscillation of eyelids with a slow downward drift and a rapid upward phase

2. Usually associated with:

       a. Convergence—seen in multiple sclerosis, Miller-Fisher syndrome, brainstem lesion

       b. Gaze shifts—damage to brainstem or cerebellum

       c. Vertical nystagmus (eg, convergence-retraction nystagmus of dorsal midbrain syndrome) (see Chapter 3, Section VI, I)

       d. Palatal myoclonus (see Chapter 3, Section VIII, G)

BIBLIOGRAPHY

Books

Jankovic J, Tolosa E, eds. *Advances in Neurology. Facial Dyskinesias.* Vol 49. New York, NY: Raven Press; 1988.

Chapters

Burde RM, Savino PJ, Trobe JD. *Clinical Decisions in Neuro-ophthalmology.* St. Louis, Mo: CV Mosby; 1992: chapter 14, 347-378.

McCord CD, Tanenbaum M, Nunnery W, eds. *Oculoplastic Surgery.* 3rd ed. New York, NY: Raven Press; 1995: 329-375.

Patel B, Weinstein GS, Anderson RL. Diagnosis and treatment of blepharospasm. In: Nesi FA, Lisman RD, Levine MR, eds. *Smith's Ophthalmic Plastic and Reconstructive Surgery.* 2nd ed. St. Louis, Mo: Mosby; 1998: 319-335.

Sibony PA, Evinger C. Anatomy and physiology of normal and abnormal eyelid position and movement. In: Miller NR, Newman NJ. *Walsh and Hoyt's Clinical Neuro-ophthalmology.* 5th ed. Vol 1. Baltimore, Md: Williams & Wilkins; 1998: 1509-1592.

Articles

Cogan DG. Myasthenia gravis: a review of the disease and a description of lid twitch as a characteristic sign. *Arch Ophthalmol.* 1965;74:217-221.

Galetta SL, Raps EC, Saito NG, Kline LB. Eyelid lag without eyelid retraction in pretectal disease. *J Neuro-ophthalmol.* 1996;16:96-98.

Janetta PJ, Abbasy M, Maroon JC, et al. Etiology and definitive microsurgical treatment of hemifacial spasm: operative techniques and results in 47 patients. *J Neurosurg.* 1977;47:321.

Jankovic J. Blepharospasm and oromandibular-laryngeal-cervical dystonia: a controlled trial of botulinum A toxin therapy. *Adv Neurol.* 1988;50:583-591.

Jordan DR, Patrinely JR, Anderson RL, et al. Essential blepharospasm and related dystonias. *Surv Ophthalmol.* 1989;34:123-132.

Russell RW. Supranuclear palsy of eyelid closure. *Brain.* 1980;103:71-82.

Schmidtke K, Buttner-Ennever JA. Nervous control of eyelid function: a review of clinical, experimental and pathological data. *Brain.* 1992;115:227-247.

Weinberg DA, Lesser RL, Vollmer TL. Ocular myasthenia: a protean disorder. *Surv Ophthalmol.* 1994;39:169-210.

Chapter 15

Headache

Patrick S. O'Connor, MD

I. **Anatomical considerations**

  A. Pain-sensitive structures within the cranium

    1. Great venous sinuses and tributaries

    2. Parts of dura at base of skull

    3. Dural and cerebral arteries at base of brain

  B. Six basic causes of intracranial headache

    1. Traction on tributary veins or displacement of great venous sinuses

    2. Traction on middle meningeal arteries

    3. Traction on large cerebral arteries or branches at the base

    4. Distension and dilation of intracranial arteries

    5. Inflammation of pain-sensitive structures

    6. Direct pressure on cranial or cervical nerves (V nerve above tentorium and IX, X, XI, and XII, and upper cervical nerves below tentorium)

  C. Extracranial sources of head pain include:

    1. Fasciae, muscles, and galea

    2. Extracranial arteries and veins of the head and neck

    3. Mucous membranes, tympanic membrane

II. **History is the key to diagnosis (95% of headache patients have a normal examination)**

  A. Where?

  B. How long?

  C. How often?

  D. Characteristics of pain (what makes it better or worse)?

  E. Accompanying signs and symptoms?

III. **Headache syndromes**

  A. Muscle contraction (tension-anxiety headache)

1. Account for 90% of all headaches
2. Acute contraction headache
   a. Emotional or physical stress
   b. Sustained contraction of neck and scalp muscles
   c. Pain, usually dull and nonthrobbing (tenderness and knotting noted in strap muscles of neck)
   d. Can be superimposed on many other headache types
3. Chronic muscle contraction headache
   a. Symptoms are "band around head," tightness, head in a vise
   b. Depression is a common denominator in these chronic, long-standing headaches

B. Migraine
   1. Migraine is a common neurologic disorder said to affect 15% to 19% of men and 25% to 29% of women. Headache is never the sole manifestation of migraine nor a necessary feature of migraine attacks. It can occur at any age, a strong family history is common as well as a history of car sickness in childhood. Frequently, erroneously attributed by the patient to "sinus" disease
   2. Migraine without aura (common migraine)
      a. Prodrome not well defined; may precede headache by hours or days and includes mood disorders, gastrointestinal distress, fatigue
      b. Photophobia, nausea and/or vomiting, and anorexia are common findings
      c. Ocular symptoms include conjunctival injection and tearing; no visual aura
   3. Migraine with aura (classic migraine)
      a. Typical syndrome
         i. Sharply defined aura, usually visual, lasting 20 to 40 minutes (Figure 15-1, see last page of book)
         ii. Visual aura: scintillating fortification scotoma, hemianopia, monocular visual loss, altitudinal field loss, tunnel vision, "heat waves"
         iii. Throbbing pain that is usually unilateral follows aura
         iv. Anorexia, nausea, noise and light sensitivity frequently accompany headache
         v. Other nonvisual symptoms such as hemiparesis, dysphasia, and cloudy thinking may precede the headache
         vi. Strong family history 80% of the time
         vii. Comprise only 20% of migraineurs
      b. Basilar artery migraine (Bickerstaff's migraine)
         i. Usually affects young women with a strong family history of migraine
         ii. Neurologic findings include bilateral visual loss, vertigo, tinnitus, hearing loss, dysesthesia, ataxia, altered consciousness
         iii. Mimics vertebrobasilar insufficiency seen in elderly patients
         iv. Distinguished by severe headache and vomiting following onset
         v. Neurologic symptoms usually clear, but permanent deficits can occur
      c. Migraine aura without headache (acephalgic migraine) denotes the occurrence of neurologic symptoms usually associated with migraine but without a headache phase

      i. Visual symptoms include scintillating scotomas, transient hemianopia, amaurosis fugax, altitudinal field loss, tunnel vision, and diplopia

      ii. Other neurologic symptoms and signs are frequently noted

      iii. Positive family history of migraine occurs in only 24% of these patients

      iv. Can present at any age, frequently confused with transient ischemic attacks when it occurs in patients over the age of 40

      v. Patients often have previous history of migraine headaches with or without aura

      vi. Diagnosis of acephalgic migraine can be made when the typical march of scintillating scotomas or other neurologic accompaniments of migraine are present. If this march is present, no further evaluation is necessary; if march is absent, the diagnosis is one of exclusion. This is one of the most common forms of migraine seen by the ophthalmologist

4. Ophthalmoplegic migraine
   a. Onset usually before age 10
   b. III nerve affected 10 to 1 over VI nerve
   c. Pupil and accommodation frequently involved
   d. Ophthalmoplegia occurs at height of headache, persisting when headache clears (may last days to weeks)
   e. Strict criteria for diagnosis
         i. Onset in first decade of life
         ii. History of typical migraine
         iii. Ophthalmoplegia ipsilateral to headache
         iv. Magnetic resonance (MR) scanning: normal or enhancement of involved ocular motor cranial nerve
         v. Some believe negative angiography also necessary

5. Retinal (ocular) migraine: transient and occasionally permanent monocular visual disturbance occurring in a young person (<40 years) with a strong history of migraine
   a. Transient visual loss may last minutes to hours
   b. May be due to temporary vasospasm of ocular circulation
   c. Rarely permanent visual deficit due to retinal or optic disc infarction
   d. Headache frequently absent during spell
   e. When no previous headache history, must rule out embolic and vasculopathic disease

6. Migraine equivalent or variant
   a. Denotes symptomatology believed to be migrainous in nature due to presumed cerebral ischemia with spreading depression, including cyclic vomiting, nausea, abdominal pain, or motion sickness in children as well as periodic fever and mood changes in children and adults
   b. Variety of disorders may occur due to presumed transient cortical dysfunction
         i. Central achromatopsia—loss of color vision
         ii. Prosopagnosia—loss of familiar face recognition
         iii. Alexia—inability to read
         iv. Transient global amnesia
         v. "Alice in Wonderland" syndrome—illusions of distortion in size and shape

7. Complications of migraine
   a. Paroxysmal neurologic defects that occur beyond headache phase, usually transient, but may be permanent
   b. Cerebral migraine: includes motor, visual, or other sensory defects
      i. Hemiplegic migraine—partial or total hemiparesis or hemiplegia (may be familial)
      ii. Transient and rarely permanent homonymous or quadrantic visual field defects
      iii. Speech disorders
      iv. Except for familial hemiplegic migraine, all patients with hemiparesis should be evaluated for a structural lesion with MR scanning

C. Cluster headache (Horton's headache, histamine cephalgia)
   1. Typically awakens patient early in the morning
   2. Severe pain in the distribution of the external carotid (frontal or frontotemporal pain)
   3. Headache accompanied by ipsilateral Horner's syndrome, lacrimation, and rhinorrhea
   4. Occasional conjunctival edema and injection
   5. Occurs in third and fourth decade with 5 to 1 male predominance
   6. Patient tends to pace floor until the pain subsides in 30 minutes to 3 to 4 hours
   7. Third-order neuron (post-ganglionic) Horner's syndrome persists in 10% of patients

D. Raeder's syndrome (painful Horner's syndrome with pain usually in V^1 distribution)
   1. Found in middle-aged or elderly males
   2. May be caused by migrainous dilatation of the internal carotid artery with compression of V^1 and sympathetic plexus in the middle cranial fossa
   3. Two types:
      a. Type one: other cranial nerves involved. Requires complete neuroradiographic investigation to rule out a parasellar mass
      b. Type two: pain in ophthalmic division with post-ganglionic Horner's only; pain may last days to weeks or months. This type can also rarely occur with fibromuscular dysplasia or spontaneous internal carotid artery dissection

E. Headache associated with brain tumor or other intracranial disease
   1. Usually appears quite suddenly
   2. May be mild or intermittent initially but progressively worsens
   3. May be worse in head down position, coughing, straining
   4. With elevated intracranial pressure, may have papilledema and VI nerve palsy
   5. Depending on causes, may have other neurologic findings

F. Other causes
   1. Hypertension should always be a diagnostic consideration
   2. Cranial arteritis
      a. New onset of headaches in patient over 60 years
      b. Bitemporal
      c. Scalp tenderness

      d. Jaw claudication

      e. Polymyalgia

      f. Visual symptoms (see Chapter 9)

   3. Sinus disease

      a. Dull, aching, and constant pain with tenderness almost universally found over the involved sinus

      b. Headaches usually aggravated by change in atmospheric pressure

      c. Many patients call migraine headaches "sinus"

   4. Headache may also be associated with temporomandibular joint dysfunction, fever, raised intracranial pressure, and ocular inflammation

   5. Headache rarely due to "eyestrain," but when due to asthenopia, pain is precipitated by eye use and relieved by rest

   6. Other causes of headache include conversion reaction, herpetic disease (zoster), and greater occipital neuralgia

BIBLIOGRAPHY

Books

Oleson J, Tfelt-Hanson P, Welch KMA. *The Headaches.* New York, NY: Raven Press; 1993.

Chapters

Burde RM, Savino PJ, Trobe JD. *Clinical Decisions in Neuro-ophthalmology.* St. Louis, Mo: Mosby-Year Book; 1992: chapter 16, 417-446.

Hupp SL. Migraine. In: Miller NR, Newman NJ, eds. *Walsh and Hoyt's Clinical Neuro-ophthalmology.* 5th ed. Vol 3. Baltimore, Md: Williams & Wilkins; 1998: 3657-3723.

Newman NM. *Neuro-ophthalmology. A Practical Text.* Norwalk, Conn: Appleton & Lange; 1992: 295-330.

Troost BT. Migraine and other headaches. In: Duane TD, ed. *Clinical Ophthalmology.* Philadelphia, Pa: Lippincott; 1994: chapter 16, 1-38.

Articles

Bickerstaff ER. Basilar artery migraine. *Lancet.* 1961;1:15-17.

Corbett JJ. Neuro-ophthalmic complications of migraine and cluster headaches. *Neurologic Clin.* 1983;1:973-995.

David RH, Daroff RB, Hoyt WF. Hemicrania, oculosynmpathetic paresis, and subcranial carotid aneurysm: Raeder's paratrigeminal syndrome (Group 2). *J Neurosurg.* 1968;29:94-96.

Fisher CM. Late-life migraine accompaniments as a cause of unexplained transient ischemic attacks. *Can J Neurol Sci.* 1980;7:9-17.

Friedman AP, Harter DH, Merritt HH. Ophthalmoplegic migraine. *Arch Neurol.* 1962;7:320-327.

Hupp SL, Kline LB, Corbett JJ. Visual disturbance of migraines. *Surv Ophthalmol.* 1989;33:221-236.

Kline LB. The neuro-ophthalmologic manifestations of spontaneous dissection of the internal carotid artery. *Sem Ophthalmol.* 1992;7:30-37.

O'Connor PS, Tredici TJ. Acephalgic migraine. Fifteen years experience. *Ophthalmology.* 1971;72:763-768.

Spector RH. Migraine. *Surv Ophthalmol.* 1984;29:193-207.

Stommel EW, Ward TN, Harris RD. MRI findings in a case of ophthalmoplegic migraine. *Headache.* 1993; 33:234-237.

Chapter 16

Carotid Artery Disease and the Eye

Milton F. White, Jr, MD

I. **General considerations**

   A. Carotid artery arteriosclerosis accounts for 20% to 50% of all strokes

   B. Cerebrovascular insufficiency is often accompanied by ocular signs and symptoms

   C. Depending upon the clinical setting, there is a spectrum of stroke risk (Table 16-1)

II. **Anatomy of the carotid system**

   A. The first major branch of the aortic arch is the innominate artery, which gives rise to the right common carotid artery

   B. The left common carotid is the second major branch of the aortic arch

   C. Each common carotid artery divides into internal and external branches at the C4 level, about 3 cm below the angle of the mandible

   D. The internal carotid artery enters the skull through the carotid canal of the temporal bone, ascends along the side of the sella turcica, forms the carotid siphon as it passes through the cavernous sinus, then emerges intracranially

   E The ophthalmic artery is its first major branch, and the internal carotid ultimately divides into the anterior and middle cerebral arteries

   F. Numerous connections between the external and internal carotid systems involve the ophthalmic artery (Figure 16-1)

   G. Third-order neuron (postganglionic) sympathetic fibers to eye, orbit, and face travel in the posterior carotid sheath

   H. Cervical portion of carotid artery is surgically accessible

III. **Ocular manifestations of carotid disease**

   A. Transient monocular blindness

      1. Amaurosis fugax—"fleeting blindness"

      2. Duration: 2 to 30 minutes

      3. Typically, a "shade" temporarily covers part or all of visual field. Other descriptions include a "dark cloud," "a film," or generalized darkening

Table 16-1

SPECTRUM OF STROKE RISK

Patient group	Risk of stroke per year (%)
No carotid disease	0.1
Asymptomatic carotid bruit	0.1 to 0.4
Amaurosis fugax	2.0
Asymptomatic carotid stenosis	2.5
Retinal infarcts, emboli	3.0
Transient cerebral ischemic attack	8.0

Reprinted with permission from Trobe JD. Carotid endarterectomy: who needs it? *Ophthalmology.* 1987;94:725-730.

4. Visual loss may include entire visual field or only half or a quadrant of the field
5. Positive visual phenomena may be described by one-third of patients
6. Amaurosis fugax associated with carotid stenosis is most commonly due to embolic disease (see below)
7. Less common pathophysiologic mechanisms include diminished blood flow (hypoperfusion) and vasospasm of the ophthalmic and/or central retinal artery
8. Occasionally, amaurosis fugax can be precipitated by exposure to bright light (retinal vascular insufficiency to photoreceptors)
9. Natural history of amaurosis fugax:
    a. Risk of permanent visual loss—1% per year
    b. Risk of stroke—2% per year (20 times higher than patient without carotid disease) (see Table 16-1)
    c. Mortality rate—2% to 4% per year
    d. Main cause of death—cardiac disease
    e. Amaurosis fugax with associated visible retinal emboli—mortality rate increases to 4% to 6% per year
10. A variety of other conditions cause transient monocular blindness (Table 16-2)

B. Retinal circulatory emboli
    1. Platelet-fibrin
        a. Fisher plugs
        b. White intra-arterial plugs lodge at bifurcations
        c. Source: internal carotid artery atheroma and ulceration
    2. Cholesterol
        a. Hollenhorst plaques
        b. Bright, orange-yellow, refractile
        c. Source: carotid and aortic atheroma
    3. Calcium
        a. Gray-white, nonrefractile
        b. Usually lodge in retinal arterioles near or on the optic disc
        c. Source: cardiac valves or aortic wall

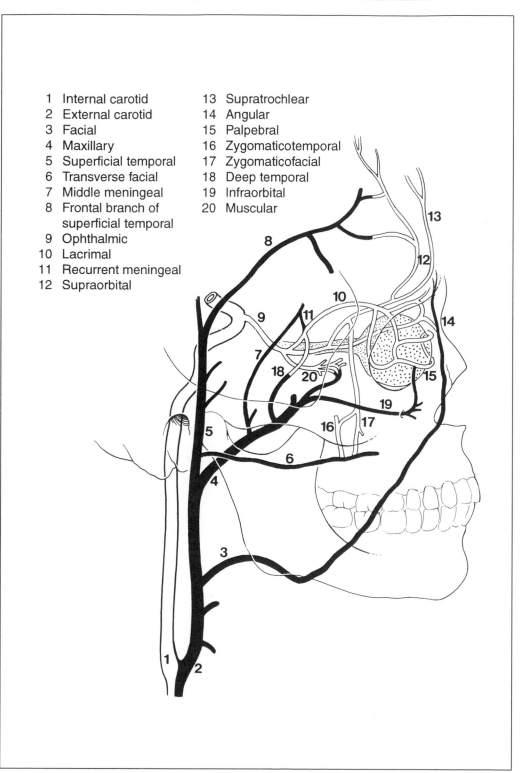

1 Internal carotid
2 External carotid
3 Facial
4 Maxillary
5 Superficial temporal
6 Transverse facial
7 Middle meningeal
8 Frontal branch of
   superficial temporal
9 Ophthalmic
10 Lacrimal
11 Recurrent meningeal
12 Supraorbital

13 Supratrochlear
14 Angular
15 Palpebral
16 Zygomaticotemporal
17 Zygomaticofacial
18 Deep temporal
19 Infraorbital
20 Muscular

Figure 16-1. Anastomotic connection between the internal and external carotid arteries. Note the key position of the ophthalmic artery (9).

Table 16-2

CONDITIONS ASSOCIATED WITH TRANSIENT MONOCULAR BLINDNESS

Intraocular

Hyphema

Glaucoma

Papilledema

Disc drusen

Congenital anomalies of the optic disc

Ischemic optic neuropathy

Intraorbital

Hemangioma

Osteoma

Intracranial

Arteriovenous malformation

Tumor

Carotid artery

Embolism

Thrombosis

Dissection

Cardiac

Embolism

Arrhythmia

Valvular disease

Hematologic

Anemia

Polycythemia

Sickle cell disease

Thrombocytosis

Other conditions

Hypertension

Hypotension

Migraine

Raynaud's phenomenon

Antiphospholipid antibodies

Modified from Seybold ME. Nonembolic sources of amaurosis fugax. In: Bernstein EF, ed. *Amaurosis Fugax.* New York, NY: Springer-Verlag; 1988: 168-173.

---

    4. Septic vegetation—bacterial endocarditis
    5. Fat—long bones
    6. Myxoma—heart
    7. Amniotic fluid—uterus
    8. Rare—mercury, air, paraffin
  C. Retinal arterial occlusion
    1. Types:
        a. Central retinal artery occlusion (CRAO)
        b. Branch retinal artery occlusion (BRAO)
    2. Central retinal artery has narrowest diameter at lamina cribrosa, where it is most vulnerable to occlusion
    3. Five major causes of CRAO:
        a. Embolization
        b. Localized atheromatous stenosis

        c. Arteritic obliteration

        d. Reduced vascular perfusion

        e. Vasospasm

4. Patient with CRAO reports painless loss of vision

5. CRAO persisting greater than 100 minutes leads to permanent loss of vision

6. Clinical findings with CRAO

        a. Segmentation of blood in retinal arterioles—"box-carring"

        b. Visible emboli in 11% to 20% of patients

        c. Axoplasmic flow stasis with retinal edema or "whitening"

        d. "Cherry-red" macular spot

        e. After several days retinal swelling subsides; loss of retinal nerve fiber layer; optic atrophy (4 to 8 weeks)

        f. Arteries may demonstrate both narrowing and sheathing

7. Clinical findings in BRAO

        a. Segmentation of blood in involved branch retinal arteriole—"box-carring"

        b. Visible emboli in 60% to 68% of patients

        c. Retinal edema localized to area of involved arteriole

        d. With resolution of retinal swelling, area of nerve fiber layer atrophy; segmental optic atrophy

8. Emergency treatment of CRAO

        a. Immediate goal is to increase perfusion and preserve flow in the CRAO:

            i. Lower intraocular pressure

            ii. Vasodilation

        b. Lower intraocular pressure: anterior chamber paracentesis, ocular massage, topical beta-blocker, systemic carbonic anhydrase inhibitor

        c. Vasodilation: breathe into paper bag, inhalation of carbogen (95% O_2, 5% CO_2), IV aminophylline, retrobulbar anesthesia

        d. All treatment modalities are empiric; none proven due to lack of controlled studies

9. Three to 10% of patients older than 50 years with CRAO have giant cell arteritis. Remember to obtain a Westergren sedimentation rate STAT!

D. Evaluation and therapy for patients with amaurosis fugax and retinal arterial occlusions

    1. Careful history searching for vascular risk factors:

        a. Hypertension

        b. Diabetes mellitus

        c. Hypercholesterolemia/hyperlipidemia

        d. Tobacco use

        e. Cardiac disease: ischemic, valvular, arrhythmia

    2. Diagnostic studies are summarized in Table 16-3

    3. Treatment

        a. Medical

            i. Reduction of vascular risk factors

            ii. Aspirin

            iii. Ticlopidine

Table 16-3

EVALUATION OF THE PATIENT WITH OCULAR ISCHEMIA

History

Physical examination
Eye
Neck (extracranial carotid artery)
Heart

Hematologic
CBC, platelet count, ESR, PT, PTT
Chemistry profile, serum lipids
ANA, FTA-Abs
Selected patients
Hypercoagulable states (protein C, S; antithrombin III; antiphospholipid antibodies)
Hyperviscosity syndromes (polycythemia; sickle cell disease)

Diagnostic procedures
Chest radiology
EKG
Carotid duplex scanning
Magnetic resonance angiography
Selected patients
Echocardiography
Carotid angiography

Modified from Carter JE. Carotid artery disease and its ocular manifestations. *Ophthalmol Clin NA.* 1992;5:425-443.

        iv. Plavix

        v. Coumadin

    b. Surgical

        i. Cardiac—if source of emboli

        ii. Carotid—North American Symptomatic Carotid Endarterectomy Trial (NASCET): endarterectomy recommended for all patients with symptomatic extracranial stenosis of 70% or greater whose medical condition does not preclude surgery (Table 16-4)

        iii. **Remember:** consider the surgical perioperative morbidity/mortality rate of your patient versus the natural history of the disease (see Table 16-1) when considering surgical intervention

E. Ischemic ocular syndrome

    1. Chronic hypoperfusion of the globe from ipsilateral or bilateral carotid occlusive disease

    2. Subdivide findings (Table 16-5)

        a. Anterior segment ischemia

        b. Hypoperfusion retinopathy

    3. Ischemic uveitis is nonresponsive to topical corticosteroid drops

    4. Hypoperfusion retinopathy, also known as venous stasis retinopathy, occurs three to four times more commonly than anterior segment ischemia

    5. Retinopathy typically located in the midperiphery

    6. Treatment

Table 16-4

HIGH-RISK FACTORS FOR CAROTID ENDARTERECTOMY PERIOPERATIVE STROKE/DEATH

Age ≥ 70 years
Refractory hypertension
Severe coronary disease
Severe obstructive pulmonary disease
Marked obesity
Recent or multiple strokes
Bilateral carotid stenosis
Distal ipsilateral carotid stenosis

Modified from Carter JE. Carotid artery disease and its ocular manifestations. *Ophthalmol Clin NA.* 1992;5:425-443.

Table 16-5

FINDINGS IN OCULAR ISCHEMIC SYNDROME

Conjunctiva
Injected vessels
Dilated episcleral vessels

Cornea
Edema

Anterior chamber
Cells, flare (ischemic uveitis)

Iris
Neovascularization
± Increased intraocular pressure

Pupil
Sluggish
Afferent defect

Lens
Cataract

Retina
Dilated arterioles
Dilated venules
Microaneurysms
Retinal hemorrhages
Neovascularization
Vitreous hemorrhage
Traction retinal detachment

    a. Ocular neovascularization requires panretinal photocoagulation
    b. Medical and surgical therapy to improve carotid artery flow to the eye
F. Horner's syndrome
    1. Rare occurrence with either atherosclerotic occlusion or dissection of the internal carotid artery
    2. Interruption of third-order neuron of sympathetic chain within carotid sheath
    3. May be associated with ipsilateral headache, neck pain, monocular blindness, stroke
G. Ocular motor cranial nerve palsies
    1. Very rare association with carotid thrombosis or dissection
    2. Ocular pain
    3. Ipsilateral blindness

4. III, IV, VI nerve palsies last 6 to 24 hours
5. Thrombosis of branches of ophthalmic artery supplying orbital branches of III, IV, IV nerves causes ophthalmoplegia; transient because collateral flow is able to restore perfusion to ocular motor nerves (see Figure 16-1)

BIBLIOGRAPHY

Books

Bernstein EF, ed. *Amaurosis Fugax.* New York, NY: Springer-Verlag; 1988.

Chapters

Burde RM, Savino PJ, Trobe JD. *Clinical Decisions in Neuro-ophthalmology.* St. Louis, Mo: Mosby-Year Book; 1992: chapter 5, 117-144.

Newman NJ. Cerebrovascular diseases. In: Miller NR, Newman NJ, eds. *Walsh and Hoyt's Clinical Neuro-ophthalmology.* Vol 3. 5th ed. Baltimore, Md: Williams & Wilkins; 1998: 3323-3656.

White MF, Kline LB. Ocular manifestations of carotid artery disease. In: Farris BK, ed. *The Basics of Neuro-ophthalmology.* St. Louis, Mo: Mosby-Year Book; 1991: 319-343.

Articles

Barnett HJM, Taylor DW, Eliasziw M, et al. North American Symptomatic Carotid Endarterectomy Trial collaborators: benefit of carotid endarterectomy in patients with moderate or severe stenosis. *N Engl J Med.* 1998;339:1415-1425.

Carter JE. Carotid artery disease and its ocular manifestations. *Ophthalmol Clin NA.* 1992;5:425-443.

Chassin MR. Appropriate use of carotid endarterectomy. *N Engl J Med.* 1998;339:1468-1471.

Cullen JR. Occult temporal arteries. A common cause of blindness in old age. *Br J Ophthalmol.* 1967;51:513-518.

Digre KB, Durean FJ, Branel DW, et al. Amaurosis fugax associated with antiphospholipid antibodies. *Ann Neurol.* 1989;25:228-232.

Fisher CM. Observation of the fundus oculi in transient monocular blindness. *Neurology.* 1959;9:333-347.

Goodwin JA, Gorelick PB, Helgason CM. Symptoms of amaurosis fugax in atherosclerotic carotid artery disease. *Neurology.* 1987;37:829-832.

Hayreh SS, Kolder HE, Weingeist TA. Central retinal artery occlusion and retinal tolerance time. *Ophthalmology.* 1980;87:75-78.

Hollenhorst RS. Significance of bright plaques in the retinal arterioles. *JAMA.* 1961;178:23-29.

Katz B, ed. Transient monocular visual loss. *Ophthalmol Clin NA.* 1996;9:323-525.

Kearns TP, Hollenhorst R. Venous-stasis retinopathy of occlusive disease of the carotid artery. *Proc Staff Mtg Mayo Clin.* 1963;38:304-312.

Kline LB. The neuro-ophthalmologic manifestations of spontaneous internal carotid artery dissection. *Sem Ophthalmol.* 1992;7:30-37.

North American Symptomatic Carotid Endarterectomy Trial Collaborators. Beneficial effect of carotid endarterectomy in symptomatic patients with high-grade carotid stenosis. *N Engl J Med.* 1991;325:445-453.

Savino PJ, Glaser JS, Cassady J. Retinal stroke: is the patient at risk? *Arch Ophthalmol.* 1977;95:1185-1189.

Trobe JD. Carotid endarterectomy: who needs it? *Ophthalmology.* 1987;94:725-730.

Wilson WB, Levengood JM, Ringel SP, et al. Transient ocular motor paresis associated with acute internal carotid artery occlusion. *Ann Neurol.* 1989;25:286-290.

Chapter 17

Hysteria and Malingering

Richard H. Fish, MD

I. **Definitions and historical perspective**

    A. Malingering: willfully misleading the existence or seriousness of a disease or disability for the purpose of a consciously desired end

        1. Duke-Elder: "Common manifestation of human weakness... wicked or lazy"

        2. Keltner: California syndrome—economic gain from visual loss. Estimated $300 million paid in 1982 for fraudulent workers' compensation claims

    B. Hysteria (Greek: "condition of the womb"): also known as conversion disorder. Subconscious expression of symptoms without demonstrable organic findings, usually involving loss or alteration of sensorimotor functions. Symptoms may have underlying symbolic meaning and are often precipitated by psychological stress or physical trauma

        1. Referred to in Egyptian papyri, writings of Hippocrates, and in the New Testament of the Bible

        2. Plato: unfulfilled uterus wandering about the body

        3. Charcot: "dissociation of vision" caused by lesion in brain

        4. Babinski: "pithiatism"; disorders caused by suggestion and cured by persuasion

        5. Freud: sexual pleasure in looking (scopophilia); results in repression of forbidden sights into the unconscious with the eyes now "at the disposal of the repressed sexual instinct and hence unable to function properly"

    C. Differentiating malingering from hysteria

        1. Can be difficult to separate; both entities form part of the spectrum of **functional or nonorganic eye disease**

        2. Malingerer will exaggerate symptoms ("blinder than the blind"), while hysterics are classically described as having "la belle indifference" to their affliction

        3. Hysterical patients tend to be cooperative; malingerers irritable and combative, especially with prolonged testing

        4. Malingering usually involves secondary gain (eg, financial reward or avoiding military service). Hysterics may receive secondary gain in the form of attention

II. Evaluation: similar for both malingering and hysteria. Learn a few tests well and be able to perform them quickly and naturally

    A. Total binocular blindness: rare, tends to occur in hysterical blindness

        1. Observation: truly blind moves cautiously, bumps into things naturally; hysteric avoids objects, "seeing unconsciously"; malingerer goes out of his or her way to bump into objects

        2. Pupillary response: easiest and single most important test

            a. Intact direct and consensual responses exclude anterior visual pathway disease (don't forget about pharmacologic mydriasis in a malingerer)

            b. In patients with vision better than NLP (no light perception), there is no consistent relationship between amount of visual loss and pupillary deficit

        3. Menace reflex: blinking to visual threat

        4. Sudden strong illumination. Difficult to suppress reflex tearing

        5. Signature: truly blind have no difficulty. Functionally blind sign their name with exaggerated illegibility

        6. Looking at hand or touching index fingers together depends on proprioception, not vision. Blind have no trouble with this; malingerers, thinking that these tasks require good vision, will perform poorly

        7. Optokinetic nystagmus: difficult but possible to suppress. Optimum response obtained when rate of succession of object is 3 to 12 per second

        8. Mirror tracking: eyes move in response to the image in a mirror as it is rocked back and forth. Mirror must be large enough to prevent patient from looking around it (approximately 33 x 67 cm)

        9. Making sudden ridiculous facial expressions. Results in "considerable loss of dignity... and residents falling into an acute fit of choking" (Thompson, 1985)

      10. Visual evoked response (VER): flash and pattern-reversal stimuli. Correlation exists between check size and level of acuity. Although difficult, it is possible to consciously alter response to pattern-reversal stimulation with convergence, meditation, and intense concentration

    B. Total monocular blindness: more common than binocular, tends to occur with malingering. Can use any of the above tests with unaffected eyes occluded

        1. Diplopia tests

            a. Suspected eye is occluded while a strong prism is held with the apex bisecting the pupil of the good eye. Patient admits to monocular diplopia. As the suspected eye is uncovered, the entire prism is placed before the good eye, producing binocular diplopia. If the patient still reports diplopia, functional blindness is revealed

            b. Have the patient walk up and down stairs with a vertical prism over the allegedly blind eye

        2. Fixation tests

            a. Ten-diopter base-out test: relies upon refixation movements to avoid diplopia. Ten-diopter base-out prism in front of a normal eye produces shift of both eyes with a refixation movement of the other eye. A truly blind eye will not refixate, and a prism placed before this eye should result in no movement of either eye

b. Vertical bar: ruler held 5 inches from the nose in between the eyes while the patient reads at near. Overlap of visual fields allows a binocular person to read across the bar without interruption. A truly monocular patient will pause to shift fixation across the bar. If the patient reads without interruption, functional blindness is confirmed. Can also use a prism in front of the suspected eye, resulting in diplopia that should interrupt reading

3. Fogging tests

    a. Both eyes are open in a phoropter; the patient begins reading the eye chart. Examiner progressively adds more plus to the good eye while the patient keeps reading. Final line read is the patient's acuity in the suspected eye

    b. Crossed cylinder technique: two strong cylindrical lenses of equal power—plus and minus—are placed at the same axis in the trial frame over the sound eye. Patient reads with both eyes open and the examiner, pretending to make an adjustment, rotates one lens 45 degrees, fogging the good eye

    c. Instill a cycloplegic agent into the unaffected eye; have the patient read at near

4. Color tests

    a. Red/green duochrome in the projector, red/green glasses worn such that the red lens covers the suspected eye. Eye behind the red lens sees letters on red and not green side of the chart; eye behind the green lens sees only letters on the green side. If the patient reads the entire line, the suspected eye is being used

    b. Red/green glasses and Worth four-dot test. Patient should see appropriate number of dots

    c. Polaroid glasses and vectographic slides: each eye sees different portions of the eye chart. If the patient reads entire line, both eyes are being utilized

5. Stereoscopic tests: stereoacuity is directly proportional to Snellen acuity—40 seconds of arc stereoacuity compatible with no worse than 20/20 Snellen acuity OU

C. Diminished vision: simulation of visual acuity less than 20/20. More difficult to detect. May be binocular or monocular. Can use most of the tests above, plus the following:

1. DKR ("doctor killing refraction") or toothpaste refraction ("squeeze it out of them"): start with 20/10 line and express disbelief that the patient could not see the huge letters on the 20/15 line, then proceed up the chart until the patient reads

2. Visual angle: varying test distances with eye chart, Landolt C rings or Tumbling E block such that the patient sees a smaller visual angle or demonstrates inconsistencies (eg, reading 20/20 letters at 10 feet is equivalent to 20/40 acuity)

3. Move the patient back and forth slightly in the chair, helping him or her "get into focus" or place combinations of lenses adding up to plano in a trial frame to help magnify the vision

III.   Conditions misdiagnosed as functional visual loss

A. Keratoconus: biomicroscopy, K readings

B. Amblyopia: look for strabismus, anisometropia

C. Early Stargardt's disease: macular examination, fluorescein angiography

D. Retinitis pigmentosa (RP) sine pigmento: ERG

E. Central serous chorioretinopathy: macular examination, fluorescein angiography

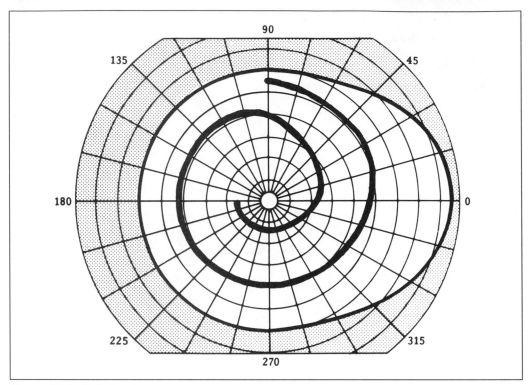

Figure 17-1. Spiraling isopters.

    F. Cystoid macular edema: ophthalmoscopy, fluorescein angiography

    G. Cone dystrophy: ERG

IV.   **Other functional eye diseases**

    A. Hysterical visual field loss

        1. Monocular visual field defects

            a. Concentric contraction with no expansion of the field at an increasing test distance (tunnel vision, see Figure 1-23 and Chapter 1 for differential diagnosis of markedly constricted visual fields)

            b. Spiraling isopters (Figure 17-1)

            c. Crossing isopters (Figure 17-2)

            d. These same visual field defects have also been reported in patients with frontal lobe tumors

            e. Monocular temporal hemianopia that persists on binocular testing (Figure 17-3)

        2. Binocular visual field defects

            a. Normal binocular perimetry: visual field performed with both eyes open measures approximately 180 degrees in width with no blind spots due to overlap of monocular fields

            b. Monocular visual field subtends approximately 150 degrees, with a greater field temporally due to unpaired temporal crescent (see Chapter 1)

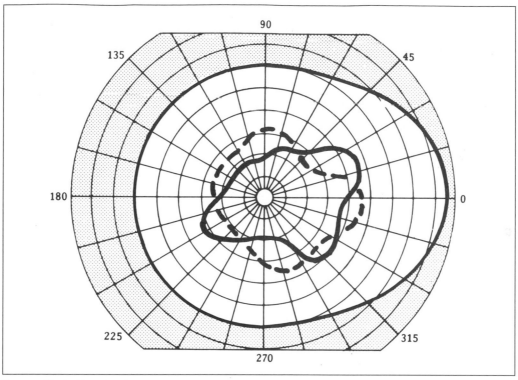

Figure 17-2. Crossing isopters.

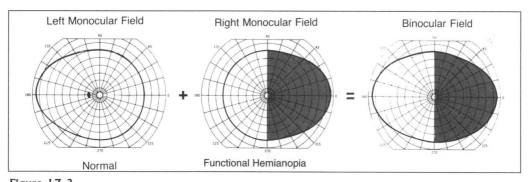

Figure 17-3.

    c. True monocular blindness: binocular perimetry demonstrates blind spot of a normal eye with loss of the temporal crescent of the blind eye (Figure 17-4)

    d. Functional monocular blindness: binocular perimetry reveals a full visual field (Figure 17-5)

    e. Hysterical bitemporal hemianopia: patients with true bitemporal hemianopia have a binocular field composed of two nasal hemifields (Figure 17-6). With functional bitemporal hemianopia, the patient claims inability to see temporally, with only a thin island of vision straddling the vertical midline (Figure 17-7)

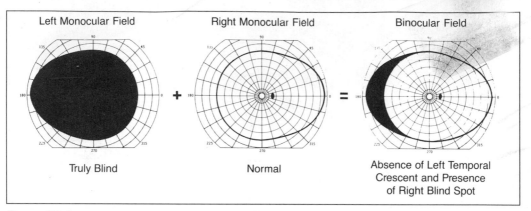

Figure 17-4.

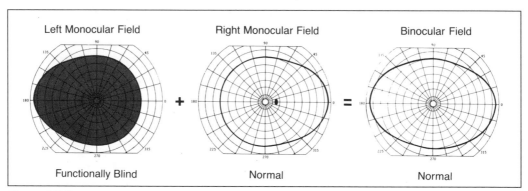

Figure 17-5.

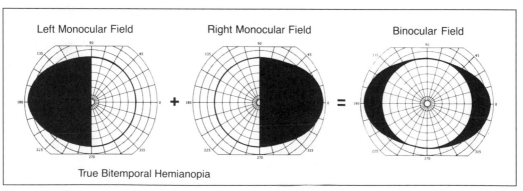

Figure 17-6.

    f. Binasal hemianopia: rare. Usually due to optic nerve or retinal disease (glaucoma, disc drusen, chronic papilledema, retinoschisis, retinal detachment, chorioretinal degeneration). Intracranial causes include basilar skull fracture, neurosyphilis, chiasmal arachnoiditis, and neoplasm. Binasal defects of organic etiology are seldom complete and rarely respect the vertical midline. If defects are complete, there is "prefixation blindness" (Figure 17-8)

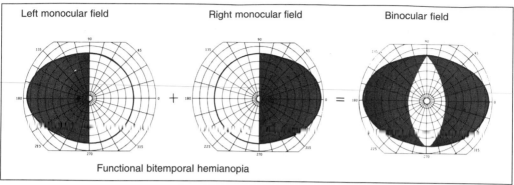

Left monocular field	Right monocular field	Binocular field

Functional bitemporal hemianopia

Figure 17-7.

       g. Caution: automated perimetry cannot differentiate functional from organic visual field loss. Malingerers can simulate neurologic field defects when tested with an automated visual field machine

B. Voluntary nystagmus (see Chapter 3)
    1. Irregular brief bursts of rapid frequency, low amplitude, horizontal pendular eye movements; actually back-to-back saccades
    2. Up to 8% of normal individuals can produce this
    3. Usually bilateral and conjugate
    4. May be associated with convergence, fluttering eyelids, blinking, or strained facial expression
    5. Oscillopsia common
    6. The initiation of nystagmus is under voluntary control, while rate, amplitude, and duration of nystagmus are not
    7. Difficult to maintain longer than 10 to 20 seconds
    8. May be familial

C. Accommodative spasm
    1. Relatively common
    2. Intermittent episodes of convergence associated with miosis, accommodation, and induced myopia
    3. Pupils constrict on attempted lateral gaze (Figure 17-9)
    4. No abduction deficit with oculocephalic (doll's head) or caloric testing
    5. May have diplopia and micropsia
    6. May be interrupted by patching or cycloplegia
    7. Differential diagnosis includes VI nerve palsy and other conditions causing limited abduction (see Chapter 4)
    8. Treatment is difficult; may involve atropine drops and bifocals

D. Monocular diplopia: usually functional cause but occasionally organic
    1. External causes: chalazion; eyelid tumor at ridge of corneal epithelium; mucus strand, vegetable fiber, or oil droplet in tear film
    2. Optical causes: irregular astigmatism; keratoconus; tilted or subluxed lens; lens clefts, vacuoles, or cataracts; gas bubbles, glass, crystals, parasite larvae in vitreous; macular cysts; epimacular membrane, central serous chorioretinopathy, diabetic macular edema causes distortion, not diplopia

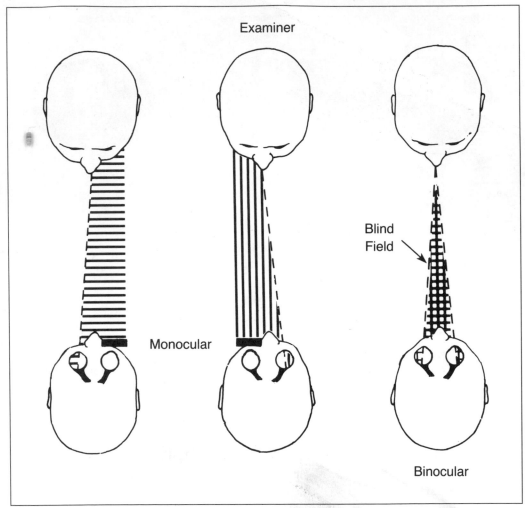

Examiner

Monocular

Blind
Field

Binocular

Figure 17-8. Binasal hemianopia. Monocular testing reveals hemianopic field defects nasal to the visual axis in each eye. With organic etiology, binocular testing confirms blindness in the area where the two nasal hemifields overlap (prefixation blindness). An object moving through this area will suddenly disappear and reappear (modified from Thompson HS. Binasal field loss. In: Thompson HS, ed. *Topics in Neuro-ophthalmology.* Baltimore, Md: Williams & Wilkins; 1979: 84).

      3. Neurologic causes: rare. Reported in pituitary tumor, tumor or hemorrhage of occipital cortex, lesions in frontal eye field controlling voluntary eye movement

      4. Transiently seen following strabismus surgery in patients with anomalous retinal correspondence

      5. Diagnosis: pinhole usually eliminates optical causes. Careful retinoscopy and biomicroscopy is essential. Contact lenses may be useful in correcting about 60% of cases of monocular diplopia

E. Voluntary blepharospasm

    1. May be unilateral or bilateral

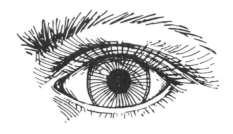
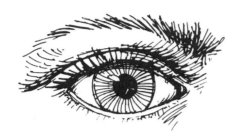

A. PRIMARY POSITION

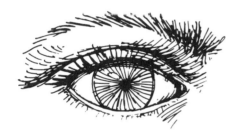
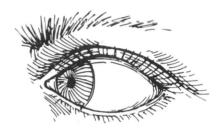

B. ATTEMPTED RIGHT GAZE
WITH ACCOMMODATIVE SPASM

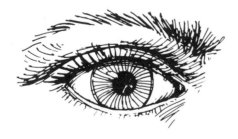
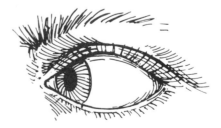

C. ATTEMPTED RIGHT GAZE
WITH RIGHT ABDUCTION DEFICIT

Figure 17-9.

2. May resemble ptosis or true blepharospasm

3. Isolated or associated with functional decreased vision or accommodative spasm

F. Hysterical asthenopia

1. Complaints of painful sensations in and around the eyes, lacrimation, photophobia

2. Inability to read without headache or eyestrain despite correction of refractive error and normal muscle balance

G. Voluntary gaze palsy

1. Infrequently seen

2. Limitation of upgaze

a. Lack of cooperation

b. Normal aging phenomenon

c. Functional etiology

d. Rule out dorsal midbrain syndrome (see Chapter 2)

3. Paralysis of horizontal gaze: one case report of a patient unable to make saccadic or pursuit movements to the left. Examiners were unable to overcome "paralysis" with oculocephalic (doll's head) testing, OKN, or mirror tracking. Also noted were convergence and miosis on attempted left gaze

H. Ocular Münchausen's syndrome

1. Deliberate deception by a patient involving fabricated medical histories, self-inflicted physical abnormalities, and self-mutilation

2. Reported ocular manifestations include voluntary nystagmus; subconjunctival hemorrhage; conjunctivitis; pharmacologic mydriasis; corneal erosion, ulcer, and alkali burn; self-induced chronic orbital cellulitis requiring exenteration; and chronic periorbital abscess

3. Psychiatric evaluation mandatory, but treatment is frequently unsuccessful

I. Hysterical chromatopsia or micropsia

V. **Treatment of functional eye disease**

A. Reassurance that the problem will get better, emphasizing positive things that the eye does well—peripheral vision, normal pupils, optic nerve, retina, etc

B. Do not use eye drops, orthoptic exercises, or spectacles. This draws attention to the eyes and undermines reassurance

C. Confrontation is rarely productive

D. Psychiatric consultation

E. "Retinal rest": hospitalized with bilateral patches and sensory deprivation (no radio, TV, visitors, etc)

VI. **Natural story of functional visual loss**

A. Twenty-seven percent of patients demonstrated a chronic course with no improvement of visual acuity (Friesen)

B. Twelve percent of patients eventually found to have macular disease (Rada)

C. Twenty-three of 42 patients (55%) continued to have functional visual loss when followed 16 to 156 months (mean: 53 months). Few were socially or economically impaired despite persistent visual loss (Kathol)

D. Seventy-two percent of 46 patients younger than 21 years of age showed improvement in functional visual field loss (Murata)

E. Beware of the patient with both organic and nonorganic disease. A follow-up study of 85 patients with a variety of hysterical conversion disorders (Slater) found that:
1. Twenty-two patients were found to have coexistent organic diseases, including generalized disease of the central nervous system
2. Two patients subsequently developed schizophrenia
3. Four patients committed suicide
4. Eight patients died of organic disease that was present at the time of diagnosis of "hysteria"

BIBLIOGRAPHY

Chapters

Freud S. The psycho-analytic view of psychogenic disturbances of vision. In: *The Standard Edition of the Complete Psychological Works of Sigmund Freud.* London: Hogarth Press; 1957: XI,211-218.

Kline LB. Techniques for diagnosis functional visual loss. In: Parrish RK, ed. *The University of Miami Bascom Palmer Eye Institute Atlas of Ophthalmology.* Boston, Mass: Butterworth-Heinemann; 2000: 493-501.

Miller NR, Keane JR. Neuro-ophthalmologic manifestations of nonorganic disease. In: Miller NR, Newman NJ, eds. *Walsh and Hoyt's Clinical Neuro-ophthalmology.* 5th ed. Vol 1. Baltimore, Md: Williams & Wilkins; 1998: 1765-1786.

Articles

Bumgartner J, Epstein CM. Voluntary alteration of visual evoked potentials. *Ann Neurol.* 1982;12:475-478.

Caplan LR, Nadelson T. Multiple sclerosis and hysteria. Lessons learned from their association. *JAMA.* 1980;24:2418-2421.

Friesen H, Mann WA. Follow-up study of hysterical amblyopia. *Am J Ophthalmol.* 1966;62:1106-1115.

Gogela LJ, Rucker CW. Psychogenic changes in the field of vision associated with tumors of the frontal lobe of the brain. *Am J Ophthalmol.* 1951;34:185-188.

Kathol RG, Cox TA, Corbett JJ, et al. Functional visual loss. II. Psychiatric aspects in 42 patients followed for 4 years. *Psychol Med.* 1983;13:315-324.

Keane JR. Hysterical hemianopia. The "missing half" defect. *Arch Ophthalmol.* 1979;97:865-866.

Keltner JL, May WN, Johnson CA, et al. The California syndrome. Functional visual complaints with potential economic impact. *Ophthalmology.* 1985;92:427-435.

Kramer KK, La Piana FG, Appleton B. Ocular malingering and hysteria: diagnosis and management. *Surv Ophthalmol.* 1979;24:89-96.

Murata M, Takahashi S. Psychogenic visual disturbances in patients under 21 years of age. *Folia Ophthalmol Jpn.* 1993;44:53-58.

Rada RT, Krill AE, Meyer GG, et al. Visual conversion reaction in children II. Followup. *Psychosomatics.* 1973;14:271-276.

Records RE. Monocular diplopia. *Surv Ophthalmol.* 1980;24:303-306.

Rosenberg PN, Krohel GB, Webb RM, et al. Ocular Münchausen's syndrome. *Ophthalmology.* 1986;93:1120-1123.

Slater E, Glithero E. A follow-up of patients diagnosed as suffering from hysteria. *J Psychosom Res.* 1965;9:9-13.

Smith CH, Beck RW, Mills RP. Functional disease in neuroophthalmology. *Neurologic Clin.* 1983;1:955-977.

Smith TJ, Baker RS. Perimetric findings in functional disorders using automated techniques. *Ophthalmology.* 1987;94:1562-1566.

Stewart JFG. Automated perimetry and malingerers. *Ophthalmology.* 1995;102:27-32.

Thompson HS. Functional visual loss. *Am J Ophthalmol.* 1985;100:209-213.

Troost BT, Troost EG. Functional paralysis of horizontal gaze. *Neurology.* 1979;29:82-85.

Veith I. Blinders of the mind: historical reflections on functional impairment of vision. *Bull Hist Med.* 1974;48:503-516.

Chapter 18

Disorders of Higher Visual Function

Christopher A. Girkin, MD

I.   **Anatomical considerations**

    A. Information concerning different aspects of visual perception is conveyed to the striate cortex through three distinct pathways: parvocellular, magnocellular, and koniocellular (see below)

    B. From the striate cortex, this information is further analyzed by several functionally distinct visual associative areas in and adjacent to the occipital lobes to further refine the incoming information (Figures 18-1 and 18-2)

    C. From these associative areas, two occipitofugal pathways project to other cortical areas involved in higher order processing of visual perceptual information (Figure 18-3)

    D. Damage to these areas may cause selective loss of isolated components of visual perception yielding an array of perceptual abnormalities that have localizing value to the clinician

II. **Overview of the visual system**

    A. Retinogeniculate pathways:

        1. Over 22 types of ganglion cells exist in the primate retina, but only three types of ganglion cells appear to be involved in visual perception and project to specific locations within the lateral geniculate nucleus (LGN)

        2. Parvocellular pathway

            a. Originates in the midget ganglion cell in the retina; these cells have small receptive fields tuned to fine spatial resolution

            b. Conveys information concerning red-green opponency

            c. Static firing system—not keyed to detect motion

            d. Ring or High Pass Resolution perimetry and spatial contrast sensitivity test this pathway

        3. Magnocellular pathway

            a. Originates in the parasol ganglion cells in the retina, which have large receptive fields and low spatial resolution

            b. Conveys information concerning motion

            c. Phasic firing system—keyed to motion detection

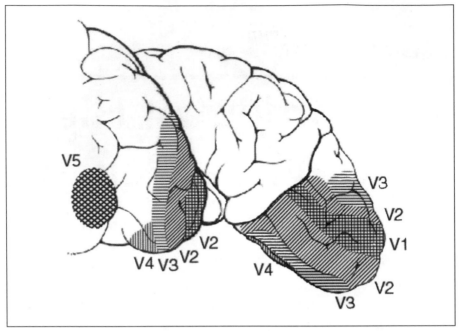

Figure 18-1. Posterior lateral view of the human visual cortex showing the clinically relevant visual associative areas. The cerebellum has been removed and the hemispheres have been separated and displaced to display medial and lateral occipital regions. V1 corresponds to the primary or striate visual cortex.

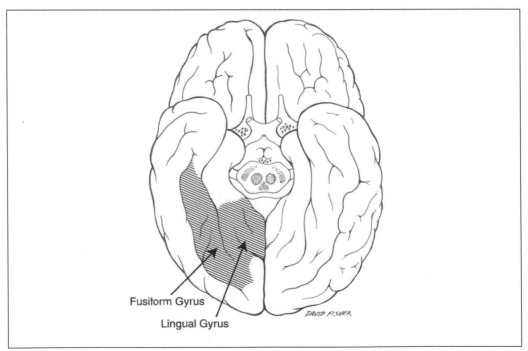

Figure 18-2. View of the ventral surface of the brain with the cerebellum removed. The posterior fusiform and lingual gyri contain the human color center.

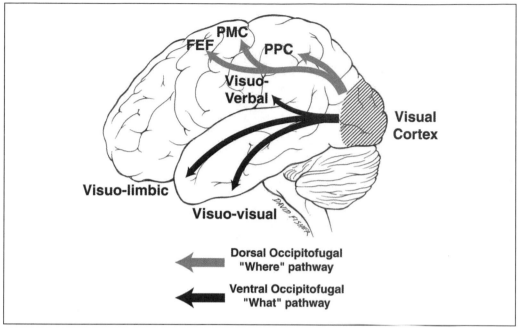

Figure 18-3. Parallel visual processing pathways in the human. The ventral, or "what," pathway begins in the striate cortex (V1) and projects to the angular gyrus for language processing, the inferior temporal lobe for object identification and limbic structures. The dorsal, or "where," pathway begins in the striate cortex and projects to the posterior parietal and superior temporal cortex, dealing with visuospatial analysis. (FEF = frontal eye field; PMC = premotor cortex; PPC = posterior parietal cortex.)

      d. Frequency doubled perimetry and motion-automated perimetry are designed to test this pathway

  4. Koniocellular pathway

      a. Originates from the bistratified ganglion cells in the retina, which have large receptive fields and low spatial resolution

      b. Conveys information concerning blue-yellow spectral opponency

      c. Short wavelength automated perimetry (SWAP) tests this pathway

B. Specialized visual cortical areas

  1. Over the past 20 years, more than 30 visual cortical areas have been isolated in macaque monkeys. These areas comprise almost 50% of the entire cortical volume

  2. The visual cortex in the macaque was initially divided into six subregions, named visual areas 1 through 6 (areas V1 to V6) which incompletely surround the striate cortex (see Figure 18-1)

  3. Area V1 is the primary visual cortex and corresponds to the striate cortex in both humans and lower primates (area 17)

  4. Areas V2 to V6 form concentric bands that incompletely surround area V1

  5. Five important cortical visual areas in man (see Figures 18-1 and 18-2)

      a. V1 or striate cortex

      b. V2 and V3—surrounds the striate cortex

Table 18-1

LESION OF ASSOCIATIVE VISUAL AREAS

1. Area V1
   a. Anton's syndrome
   b. Blindsight
   c. Riddoch's phenomenon
   d. Visual ataxia
2. Areas V2 and V3
   a. Quadrantic homonymous hemianopia
3. Area V4
   a. Cerebral achromatopsia
4. Area V5
   a. Akinetopsia

   c. V4—in the ventromedial occipital lobe involved in color perception

   d. V5—in the lateral occipital lobe involved in motion perception

6. Damage to these areas may yield a variety of visual disturbances (Table 18-1)

C. Two occipitofugal pathways convey information from the occipital lobe to more anterior visual associative areas (see Figure 18-3)

1. Dorsal occipitofugal pathway or "where" pathway
   a. Projections involved in visuospatial analysis, in the localization of objects in visual space, and in modulation of visual guidance of movements toward these objects
   b. Begins in V1 and projects through V2 and V3 to V5. From V5, this pathway continues to the parietal and superior temporal cortex
   c. Lesions of this pathway cause visuospatial disorders, such as simultagnosia, optic ataxia, acquired oculomotor apraxia, and hemispatial neglect

2. Ventral occipitofugal pathway or "what" pathway
   a. Projections involved in processing the physical attributes of a visual image that are important to the perception of color, shape, and pattern
   b. Information is crucial for object identification and object-based attention and provides visual information to areas involved in visual identification, language processing, memory, and emotion
   c. Originates in V1 and projects through V2 and V4 to specific inferior temporal cortical areas, the angular gyrus, and limbic structures
   d. Lesions in this pathway may cause a variety of associative defects including visual alexia and anomia, visual agnosia, visual amnesia, and visual hypoemotionality

III. Syndromes associated with damage to the striate cortex (area V1)

A. Anton's syndrome
   1. Definition: denial of blindness, which usually occurs following bilateral damage to the striate cortex
   2. Occasionally seen with prechiasmal blindness

3. Possible causes:
   a. Damage to higher cognitive centers
   b. Psychiatric denial
   c. Disruption of pathways from visual areas to cerebral regions involved with conscious awareness

B. Blindsight
   1. Definition: unconscious rudimentary visual perception that may persist in blind patients following lesions to the visual cortex
   2. Multiple levels of preserved function
      a. Subcortical (reflexive) blindsight:
         i. Preserved visual-neuroendocrine response due to retino-hypothalamic connections
         ii. Preservation of the photic blink reflex
         iii. Preservation of OKNs reported in one patient with cortical blindness
      b. Higher level preserved visual responses in a blind hemifield
         i. Detection of stimulus presence, type, orientation, motion, and wavelength has been described
   3. Possibly due to pathways through the superior colliculus that bypass the damaged striate cortex, or due to connections between the lateral geniculate nucleus to extrastriatal visual cortical areas
   4. While these residual abilities may be enhanced with practice, the role of blindsight in visual rehabilitation is controversial

C. Riddoch phenomenon (statokinetic dissociation)
   1. Definition: preservation of perception of motion in an otherwise blind hemifield
   2. Possible causes:
      a. Activation of extrastriate areas (V5)
      b. Residual island of function in the striate cortex
      c. Lateral summation of moving images (may be seen in normals)
   3. Clinically, the presence of Riddoch's phenomena in a hemianopic defect following an occipital stroke is a good prognostic sign that the visual field will improve

D. Visual ataxia
   1. Definition: patients with homonymous hemianopia from occipital lobe lesions may experience loss of balance with the sensation of falling toward their blind hemifield
   2. Patients have normal vestibular responses, and the "visual ataxia" is thought to be due to unopposed input from the contralateral intact visual cortex

IV. **Syndromes caused by damage to the parastriate and peristriate visual cortex (V2 and V3)**

A. Quadrantic homonymous hemianopia that respects the horizontal meridian may occur with lesions of V2 and V3 based on magnetic resonance imaging (MRI) correlations; however, this has not been corroborated in animal models

V. **Syndromes caused by damage to the human color center**

A. Cerebral achromatopsia
   1. Definition: loss of color perception due to damage to the ventromedial occipital cortex, posterior lingual, and fusiform gyri (see Figure 18-2)

Table 18-2

CAUSES OF CENTRAL ACHROMATOPSIA

1. Bilateral posterior cerebral artery infarction
2. Metastatic tumor involving the ventromedial occipital cortex
3. Posterior cortical dementia
4. Herpes simplex encephalitis involving the ventromedial occipital cortex
5. Seizure disorder (transient)
6. Migraine (transient)
7. Vertebrobasilar insufficiency (transient)

---

    2. Etiology (Table 18-2)

    3. Bilateral lesions may cause complete achromatopsia; unilateral lesions will cause hemiachromatopsia

    4. Often associated with superior visual field defects and disorders of the ventral occipitofugal pathway (see below)

VI. Syndromes caused by damage to area V5

  A. Akinetopsia

    1. Definition: loss of perception of visual motion with preservation of the perception of other modalities of vision, such as form, texture, and color

    2. Caused by bilateral lesions of the ventrolateral occipital gyri (see area V5 in Figure 18-1)

      a. Only two cases due to cerebral infarctions following sagittal sinus thrombosis have been extensively studied

      b. Subtle deficits in motion processing have been demonstrated in the contralateral hemifield in patients with unilateral damage to this area

VII. Syndromes of the dorsal occipitofugal pathway in humans

  A. Simultagnosia

    1. Definition: failure to integrate multiple elements of a visual scene into one global image

    2. Patients with simultagnosia can only attend to one element of a visual scene at a time and describe only fragments of a picture, despite intact visual fields

    3. The cookie theft picture is an excellent test for simultagnosia (Figure 18-4)

    4. Due to lesions of the posterior parietal cortex (PPC)

      a. Stroke (especially watershed infraction)

      b. Tumors

      c. Encephalitis

      d. Alzheimer's disease

      e. Posterior cortical dementia

  B. Optic ataxia

    1. Definition: a disorder of visual guidance of movements in which visual inputs are disconnected from the motor systems; thus, patients with an intact field reach for targets as if they were blind

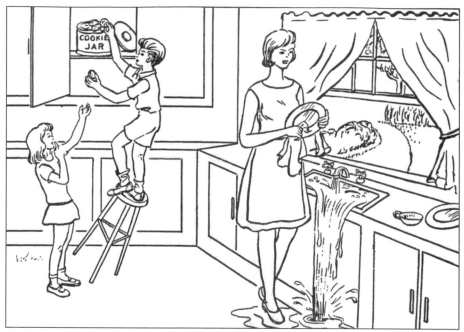

Figure 18-4. The "cookie theft picture," modified from the Boston Diagnostic Aphasia Examination. This picture contains a balance of information among the four visual field quadrants. A patient is asked to describe the events in the picture, a task that requires assimilation of the entire visual scene.

2. Etiology: a complex sensory-motor network involving the PPC (posterior parietal cortex), PMC (premotor cortex), motor areas, ventromedial cortical areas, and subcortical structures, such as the cerebellum, that modulate the control of visually guided limb movement. Any lesion that disrupts this network can cause optic ataxia

3. As a rule, lesions of the superior parietal cortex are more likely to damage areas involved with limb guidance, whereas inferior parietal lesions are more likely to affect visual attention and thus produce neglect syndromes

C. Acquired oculomotor apraxia (spasm of fixation)
    1. Definition: loss of voluntary eye movements with persistence of fixation on a target. In contrast to true ocular motor apraxia seen in childhood, saccades are easily made to peripheral targets in the absence of a fixation target
    2. Etiology: damage to the frontal eye field (FEF) inhibits the release of fixation

D. Hemispatial (hemifield) neglect
    1. Definition: a visuospatial disorder in which patients are unable to attend to stimuli presented into the left hemifield, despite full visual fields
    2. Caused by damage to a network in the right hemisphere that controls visuospatial attention to both hemispheres. These areas include:
        a. PPC—builds the sensory representation of extrapersonal space
        b. FEF—plans and initiates exploratory movements
        c. Cingulate gyrus—provides motivational potential

3. Hemispatial neglect may appear as a left homonymous hemianopia on double simultaneous confrontational field testing. Presenting stimuli to one side at a time will reveal intact areas in the left visual field that are masked with bilateral testing

4. Since the right cerebral hemisphere may mediate attention in both hemifields, right-sided hemineglect does not occur with left hemispheric lesions

E. Visual allesthesia

   1. Definition: a disorder of visuospatial perception in which the retinotopic visual field is rotated, flipped, or even inverted

   2. Causative lesion may disturb the integration of visual and otolithic inputs at the level of the medulla or at the site of integration in the posterior parietal cortex

   3. Etiology (Table 18-3)

VIII. Lesions of the ventral occipitofugal pathway in humans

A. Visual-verbal disconnection

   1. Definition: these syndromes are due to disconnection of visual input to areas in the dominant angular gyrus, which deals with language processing; thus, patients have difficulty naming objects from sight

   2. Etiology: most commonly seen with left occipital infarctions that also damages fibers crossing in the splenium of the corpus collosum carrying visual information from the right hemisphere to left-sided language areas

   3. Types:

      a. Alexia without agraphia—loss of the ability to read with preservation of writing ability

      b. Color anomia—loss of the ability to name colors with preservation of color matching (ie, color perception is normal)

      c. Optic anomia—generalized deficit in the ability to name visual objects or categories of objects

B. Visual-visual disconnection

   1. Definition: these syndromes develop due to disconnection of visual information from occipital areas to areas within the temporal lobe involved in object identification

   2. Etiology: usually results from bilateral damage to the inferior portions of the occipitotemporal cortex, notably the lingual and fusiform gyri

   3. Types:

      a. Prosopagnosia—loss of the ability to visually identify previously familiar faces. Identification by other sensory (eg, voice, mannerisms) modalities remain intact

      b. Associative object agnosia—a generalized loss of object identification that often affects multiple categories of objects (eg, cars, animals, faces)

C. Visual-limbic disconnection

   1. Definition: these syndromes develop due to disconnection of visual information from limbic structures involved in memory and emotions

   2. Etiology: due to ventral occipitotemporal lesions that damage connections to limbic structures

Table 18-3

ETIOLOGY OF VISUAL HALLUCINATIONS AND ILLUSIONS

I. Visual hallucinations
    A. Psychiatric disorders
        1. Schizophrenia
        2. Narcolepsy
        3. Psychotic depression and mania
    B. Neurologic disorders
        1. Alzheimer's dementia
        2. Epilepsy
        3. Stroke (via release hallucination of seizures)
    C. Complex multimodal peduncular hallucinations (thalamic infarction)
    D. Metabolic derangements
        1. Alcohol withdrawal
    E. Drugs
        1. Prescription: indomethacin, digoxin, bupropion, vincristine, cyclosporine, lithium, lidocaine, dopamine, topical homatropine, scopolamine, atropine, withdrawal of baclofen
        2. Hallucinogens: marijuana, PCP, psilocybin, mescaline, LSD, 3,4-methylenedioxymethamphetamine (Ecstasy), nutmeg
    F. Release hallucinations (Charles Bonnet syndrome)
    G. Visual migraines
II. Palinopsia
    A. Cerebral lesions
        1. Right parieto-occipital area
        2. Bilateral and left-sided lesions have been reported
        3. Temporal and medial occipital lobe lesions
    B. Drugs
        1. Mescaline—occasionally permanent
        2. LSD—occasionally permanent
        3. 3,4-methylenedioxymethamphetamine (Ecstasy)—occasionally permanent
        4. Clomiphene
        5. Trazodone
        6. Interleukin-2
    C. Metabolic disorders
        1. Nonketotic hyperglycemia
    D. Psychiatric disorders
        1. Creutzfeldt-Jakob disease
III. Cerebral polyopia
    A. Dominant or nondominant parietal or parieto-occipital lesion
    B. Occipital lobe injury
    C. Encephalitis
    D. Seizure
    E. Multiple sclerosis
    F. Migraine
    G. Tumor
IV. Visual allesthesia
    A. Wallenberg's lateral medullary syndrome
    B. Lesion of the posterior parietal cortex
        1. Infarction
        2. Neoplasm
        3. Trauma
        4. Infection
        5. Multiple sclerosis
        6. Migraine (transient)
        7. Seizure (transient)

3. Types:

  a. Visual amnesia—modality-specific disorder in which patients are unable to learn new visual objects, patterns, and faces or to remember visual surroundings

  b. Visual hypoemotionality—a rare syndrome in which emotional responses to visual stimuli are blunted or absent

IX. **Visual hallucinations and illusions**

  A. Of the many etiologies of hallucinations and illusions (see Table 18-3), the following four categories are of the most importance to the ophthalmologist

  1. Release hallucinations (Charles Bonnet syndrome)

    a. Definition: hallucinations that frequently occur in patients who lose vision in both eyes regardless of the location of the causative lesion or lesions

    b. May be simple (flashes of light, shapes) or complex (people, objects)

    c. Patients are psychiatrically normal and usually not disturbed by the hallucinations

    d. Occurs in 11% to 13% of blind patients

    e. Worsens with social isolation

    f. No clear treatment

  2. Visual migraines (see Chapter 15)

  3. Visual seizures

    a. Visual seizures involving the occipital or occasionally the temporal lobe may cause unformed hallucinations similar to those experienced during a classic migraine attack

    b. Temporal and rarely occipital lobe seizures may cause formed visual hallucinations, thus mimicking Charles Bonnet syndrome

    c. Distinguishing seizures from migraine is usually possible by careful history; however, seizure monitoring may be needed in some cases

    d. Characteristics of visual seizures:

      i. Usually lack the typical history of migraines

      ii. Atypical frequency and duration of hallucinations

      iii. Exhibit other seizure phenomena, such as eye deviation or rapid blinking

  4. Visual perseveration

    a. Definition: the pathologic persistence or recurrence of a previously seen visual image

    b. Types:

      i. Palinopsia

        a. Definition: the preservation in time of a previously viewed image

        b. Patients report seeing a previously viewed image immediately after it was seen or occasionally several minutes later

        c. Usually associated with an homonymous field defect and occurs in the affected portion of the field

        d. Etiology (see Table 18-3)

      ii. Cerebral polyopia

        a. Definition: the preservation in space of an image (ie, seeing two or more images)

  b. Unlike diplopia, due to optic aberrations; images are equal in clarity

  c. Homonymous field defects are often present

  d. Etiology (see Table 18-3)

BIBLIOGRAPHY

Chapters

Lessel S. Higher disorders of visual function: negative phenomena. In: Glaser J, Smith J, eds. *Neuro-ophthalmology.* Vol 8. St. Louis, Mo: Mosby; 1975: 3-4.

Rizzo M, Barton J. Central disorders of visual function. In: Miller NR, Newman, NJ, eds. *Walsh and Hoyt's Clinical Neuro-ophthalmology.* 5th ed. Vol 1. Baltimore, Md: William & Wilkins; 1998: 387-483.

Articles

Barrett AM, Beversdorf DQ, Crucian GP, Heilman KM. Neglect after right hemisphere stroke: a smaller floodlight for distributed attention. *Neurology.* 1998;51:972-978.

Bauer RM. Visual hypoemotionality as a symptom of visual-limbic disconnection in man. *Arch Neurol.* 1982;39:702-708.

Dacey DM, Lee BB. The "blue-on" opponent pathway in primate retina originates from a distinct bistratified ganglion cell type. *Nature.* 1994;367:731-735.

Damasio AR, Damasio H. The anatomic basis of pure alexia. *Neurology.* 1983;33:1573-1583.

Damasio AR, Damasio H, Van Hoesen GW. Prosopagnosia: anatomic basis and behavioral mechanisms. *Neurology.* 1982;32:331-341.

Desimone R, Schein SJ, Moran J, Ungerleider LG. Contour, color and shape analysis beyond the striate cortex. *Vision Res.* 1985;25:441-452.

Farah MJ. Agnosia. *Curr Opin Neurobiol.* 1992;2:162-164.

Hausser CO, Robert F, Giard N. Balint's syndrome. *Can J Neurol Sci.* 1980;7:157-161.

Heywood CA, Gadotti A, Cowey A. Cortical area V4 and its role in the perception of color. *J Neurosci.* 1992;12:4056-4065.

Holroyd S, Rabins PV, Finkelstein D, et al. Visual hallucinations in patients with macular degeneration. *Am J Psychiatry.* 1992;149:1701-1706.

Jacobs L. Visual allesthesia. *Neurology.* 1980;30:1059-1063.

Manford M, Andermann F. Complex visual hallucinations. Clinical and neurobiological insights. *Brain.* 1998;121:1819-1840.

Nobre AC, Sebestyen GN, Gitelman DR, et al. Functional localization of the system for visuospatial attention using positron emission tomography. *Brain.* 1997;120:515-533.

Schiller PH, Logothetis NK, Charles ER. Role of the color-opponent and broad-band channels in vision. *Vis Neurosci.* 1990;5:321-346.

Siatkowski RM, Zimmer B, Rosenberg PR. The Charles Bonnet syndrome. Visual perceptive dysfunction in sensory deprivation. *J Clin Neuro-ophthalmol.* 1990;10:215-218.

Stoerig P, Cowey A. Blindsight in man and monkey. *Brain.* 1997;120: 535-559.

Tootell RB, Taylor JB. Anatomical evidence for MT and additional cortical visual areas in humans. *Cereb Cortex.* 1995;5:39-55.

Zeki SM. Representation of central visual fields in prestriate cortex of monkey. *Brain Res.* 1969;14: 271-291.

Zeki S, Ffytche DH. The Riddoch syndrome: insights into the neurobiology of conscious vision. *Brain.* 1998;121:25-45.

Zeki S, Watson JD, Lueck CJ, et al. A direct demonstration of functional specialization in human visual cortex. *J Neurosci.* 1991;11:641-649.

Chapter 19

The Phakomatoses: Neurocutaneous Disorders

Angela R. Lewis, MD

I. **The phakomatoses defined**

    A. The phakomatoses are a group of disorders characterized by hamartomas of the skin, central nervous system, eye, and visceral organs

    B. Hamartomas are abnormal proliferations of mature cells normally found in the involved organ

II. **Neurofibromatosis type 1 (NF1)**

    A. Also known as von Recklinghausen's neurofibromatosis or peripheral neurofibromatosis

    B. NF1 occurs in approximately 1 in 3000 persons

    C. Genetics

        1. NF1 may be inherited as an autosomal dominant trait; 50% of cases are due to spontaneous mutations

        2. The NF1 gene is located on chromosome 17 (17q12-22). The gene has 100% penetrance but is highly variable in its expression

        3. The NF1 gene produces a protein called neurofibromin, which negatively regulates the oncoprotein ras, which is a tumor suppressor gene

        4. Mutations of the NF1 gene results in a loss of neurofibromin, which leaves the ras unopposed to stimulate cell growth

    D. Cutaneous lesions

        1. Café-au-lait spots are found in 99% of patients with NF1

            a. Flat hyperpigmented lesions

            b. Present at birth and increase in size and number with time

            c. Distributed randomly over the body but do not occur on the scalp, eyebrows, palms, or soles

            d. Histology: hyperpigmentation of the basal cell layer of the epithelium

2. Freckles are found in 81% of patients with NF1

   a. Hyperpigmentation of the groin, axilla, inframammary regions, and other intertriginous areas

   b. Usually present by age 6

3. Neurofibromas are benign tumors of the peripheral nerves

   a. Composed of axons, Schwann cells, and fibroblasts

   b. Localized (isolated) neurofibromas compose 80% to 90% of neurofibromas found in NF1

      i. Circumscribed lesion

      ii. Uncommon before age 6; will increase in size and number with age

   c. Plexiform neurofibromas compose 10% to 20% of neurofibromas in NF1

      i. Congenital

      ii. Extensive interdigitation into surrounding tissue

      iii. Associated with soft tissue hypertrophy

      iv. Rarely undergoes malignant transformation

E. Ocular lesions

   1. Lisch nodules

      a. Melanocytic hamartoma

      b. Tan, brown, or yellow domed-shaped lesions that protrude from the iris surface

      c. Uncommon prior to age 6, but increases in number with age

      d. Do not cause visual symptoms

   2. Eyelid

      a. Café-au-lait spots

      b. Neurofibromas—both isolated and plexiform. Plexiform neurofibromas of the upper eyelid are associated with defects of the sphenoid bone and with congenital glaucoma

   3. Orbit

      a. Orbital neurofibromas

      b. Defects in the sphenoid wing—may cause pulsating proptosis

   4. Optic nerve glioma (see Chapter 10)

      a. Predominant intracranial neoplasm in NF1. Occurs in 15% of patients with NF1

      b. Grade 1 pilocytic astrocytoma

      c. Occurs predominantly in young children; most optic nerve gliomas are diagnosed by age 6

      d. Fifty percent of patients with optic nerve and chiasmal gliomas will experience ophthalmologic problems: proptosis, strabismus, loss of visual acuity, papilledema

      e. Gliomas may involve the hypothalamus, leading to endocrine abnormalities (eg, precocious puberty, diabetes insipidus)

      f. Magnetic resonance (MR) scanning essential in demonstrating optic nerve, chiasm, optic tract, and thalamic/basal ganglia/cerebellar involvement. Optic nerve and chiasmal gliomas are diagnosed by MRI. On T_2 images, one sees a fusiform enlargement of the optic nerve

        g. Few patients with symptomatic gliomas will require treatment, whether by surgery, radiation, or chemotherapy

        h. Visual pathway gliomas may remain stable, enlarge, or regress (post-biopsy or spontaneously)

    5. Corneal nerves may be enlarged in NF1

    6. Retinal lesions are uncommon and nonspecific. Patients may have a combined hamartoma of the retina and retinal pigment epithelium (RPE) or an astrocytic hamartoma

F. Central nervous system lesions

    1. Tumors of the central nervous system are common

        a. Optic pathway glioma

        b. Brainstem glioma

        c. Schwannoma

        d. Meningioma

    2. Acqueductal stenosis

    3. Macrocephaly

    4. Headaches

    5. Seizures

    6. Impaired intellect

G. Visceral lesions

    1. Increased risk for malignancies

        a. Neurofibrosarcoma

        b. Malignant myeloid disorders

        c. Rhabdomyosarcoma

        d. Wilm's tumor

        e. Pheochromocytoma

    2. Skeletal abnormalities

        a. Short stature

        b. Pseudoarthrosis

        c. Scoliosis

    3. Hypertension may be secondary to a pheochromocytoma or renal artery stenosis

H. Diagnostic criteria: must have at least two of the following to make a diagnosis of NF1

    1. Six or more café-au-lait spots. Must measure at least 5 mm in prepubertal individuals and at least 15 mm in postpubertal individuals

    2. Two or more neurofibromas of any type or one plexiform neurofibroma

    3. Axillary or inguinal freckling

    4. Optic nerve glioma

    5. Two or more Lisch nodules

    6. Distinctive osseous lesions, such as sphenoid dysplasia or cortical thinning

    7. A first-degree relative with NF1 by the above criteria

III. Neurofibromatosis type 2 (NF2)

A. Also known as bilateral acoustic neurofibromatosis or central neurofibromatosis

B. NF2 is seen in 1 in 50,000 persons

C. Genetics
    1. NF2 is inherited as an autosomal dominant trait
    2. The NF2 gene is located on chromosome 22 (22q12). It is believed to be a tumor suppressor gene
    3. The NF2 gene produces a protein called schwannomin or merlin

D. Cutaneous lesions are uncommon. Rarely, patients will have a few (less than six) café-au-lait spots or peripheral neurofibromas

E. Ocular lesions
    1. Posterior subcapsular cataract
    2. Epiretinal membrane
    3. Combined hamartoma of the RPE and retina

F. Central nervous system lesions
    1. Bilateral vestibular schwannomas are the hallmark of this syndrome
        a. Typically present in the third decade of life
        b. Symptoms include progressive hearing loss, tinnitus, and vertigo
        c. Histology: schwannomas are benign tumors arising from Schwann cells
    2. Schwannomas of other cranial nerves, and spinal and peripheral nerves
    3. Meningiomas: optic nerve sheath, intracranial, intraspinal
    4. Gliomas
    5. Ependymomas

G. To diagnose NF2, patients must meet one of these criteria:
    1. Bilateral VIII nerve schwannomas
    2. A first-degree relative with NF2 and a unilateral VIII nerve mass
    3. A first-degree relative with NF2 and two of the following lesions: neurofibroma, meningioma, glioma, schwannoma, or a posterior subcapsular lenticular opacity

IV. Alternate forms of neurofibromatosis

A. Conditions showing some of the classic features of either condition (NF1 or NF2) but not in a typical manner

B. Alternate forms of NF1
    1. Segmental neurofibromatosis: patients have manifestations of NF1 limited to one or more areas of the body
    2. Familial café-au-lait spots: patients only have café-au-lait spots
    3. Familial spinal neurofibromatosis: patients have multiple neurofibromas along the spinal canal and café-au-lait spots

C. Schwannomatosis is an alternate form of NF2. The schwannomas are confined to the skin and spine. The VIII cranial nerves are spared

V. Tuberous sclerosis (TS)

A. Syndrome also known as Bourneville's disease

B. Incidence is estimated at 1:6000 to 1:10,000 persons

C. Genetics
    1. TS is inherited as an autosomal dominant trait, but 66% of cases represent spontaneous mutations
    2. Two distinct genes can cause TS: TSC1 and TSC2

    a. The TSC1 gene is on chromosome 9 (9q34) and encodes a protein called hamartin

    b. The TSC2 gene is on chromosome 16 (16p13) and encodes the protein tuberin

    c. Both genes are believed to be tumor suppressor genes

    d. Each gene is associated with approximately 50% of TS cases

    e. Both genes cause a similar clinical phenotype

D. Cutaneous lesions

  1. Adenoma sebaceum appears in 75% of patients with TS

    a. Reddish-brown papular rash in the malar region

    b. Histologically, these lesions are angiofibromas. They consist of vascular, fibrous, and dermal tissue elements

  2. Mountain-Ashleaf spots are seen in 90% of patients with TS

    a. Hypomelanotic macules

    b. Can be present at birth

    c. Best seen with ultraviolet light (Wood's lamp)

  3. Subungual/periungual fibromas are seen in 25% of TS patients

    a. Angiofibromas of the nail

    b. More common on toenails than fingernails

  4. Shagreen patches are seen in 20% of TS patients

    a. Connective tissue hamartoma

    b. Gross appearance: area of thickened skin, usually over the lumbosacral region

E. Ocular lesions

  1. Retinal astrocytic hamartoma

    a. Present in 75% of TS patients

    b. Multiple lesions are often found in one eye

    c. Twenty-five percent of patients will have bilateral lesions

    d. Rarely affects vision

    e. Three types of astrocytic hamartoma

      i. Type 1—flat, smooth, and semitranslucent

      ii. Type 2—opaque, nodular, elevated, and calcified

      iii. Type 3—combination of types 1 and 2

  2. Patches of RPE depigmentation

  3. Angiofibroma of the eyelids and conjunctiva

F. Central nervous system lesions

  1. Cortical tubers (hamartomas)

    a. Alterations in cerebral cortex pattern; affected gyri are enlarged and hardened

    b. Disruptions in cerebral cortical cellular pattern leads to seizures and mental retardation. Size and number of tubers positively correlate with the level of cognitive impairment and severity of seizures in patients

  2. Subependymal nodules

    a. Irregular nodules that protrude into the ventricles from the subependymal layer and often calcify

    b. Often enlarge and are then referred to as giant-cell astrocytomas

    c. May enlarge to cause obstructive hydrocephalus

G. Visceral lesions
1. Lymphangiomyomatosis affects the lung parenchyma
   a. Occurs in 1% to 6% of cases and only in women with TS
   b. Can cause spontaneous pneumothorax and respiratory failure
   c. Treatment includes hormonal therapy and lung transplantation
2. Renal system
   a. Angiomyolipomas are composed of abnormal blood vessels, smooth muscle, and adipose tissue. These renal tumors are seen in 80% of patients with TS
   b. Renal cysts are seen 15% to 20% of the time
   c. Renal cell carcinoma occurs in 2% of patients
3. Rhabdomyomas of the heart are common, seen in 67% of patients
   a. Rhabdomyomas are usually clinically silent
   b. These lesions decrease in size and may disappear over time
4. Sclerosis of the calvarium and spine occur in 40% of TS patients
5. Pitting of tooth enamel is common

H. Diagnostic criteria
- Definite TS: either two major features or one major feature plus two minor features
- Probable TS: one major feature plus one minor feature
- Suspect TS: either one major feature or two minor features
1. Major features
   a. Facial angiofibromas or forehead plaque
   b. Nontraumatic ungual or periungual fibroma
   c. Hypomelanotic macules (three or more)
   d. Shagreen patch
   e. Cortical tuber
   f. Subependymal nodule
   g. Subependymal giant cell astrocytoma
   h. Multiple retinal nodular hamartomas
   i. Cardiac rhabdomyoma
   j. Lymphangiomyomatosis
   k. Renal angiomyolipoma
2. Minor features
   a. Multiple randomly distributed pits in dental enamel
   b. Hamartomatous rectal polyps
   c. Bone cysts
   d. Cerebral white matter radial migration lines
   e. Gingival fibromas
   f. Nonrenal hamartoma
   g. Retinal achromic patch
   h. "Confetti" skin lesions
   i. Multiple renal cysts

VI. **Von Hippel-Lindau disease (VHL)**
A. Also known as angiomatosis of the retina and cerebellum

B. VHL occurs in 1 in 36,000 persons

C. Genetics

1. VHL is inherited as an autosomal dominant trait with incomplete penetrance
2. The VHL gene is on chromosome 3 (3p26). It is a tumor suppressor gene

D. There are no cutaneous lesions

E. Ocular lesion—retinal hemangioblastoma

1. Usually the first manifestation of VHL; can be missed in its early stages due to peripheral location and small size
2. Stages of a retinal hemangioblastoma
   a. Stage 1—preclassical: lesion is small and without feeder vessels
   b. Stage 2—classical: lesion takes on a globular shape and feeder vessels are evident
   c. Stage 3—marked by extravasation of lipid and plasma
   d. Stage 4—reached if a retinal detachment occurs
   e. Stage 5—marked by blindness secondary to retinal detachment, glaucoma, or persistent uveitis
3. Fifty percent of patients will have bilateral eye disease. Sixty percent will have multiple lesions in one eye. Fifty percent will have severe visual loss
4. Histologically, hemangioblastomas are composed of capillaries and glial cells
5. This lesion can be treated with photocoagulation or cryotherapy

F. Central nervous system lesions

1. Hemangioblastoma
   a. Most often located in the cerebellum (52%), but can occur in the spinal cord (44%) and brainstem (18%)
   b. Usually asymptomatic until the third decade of life. Patients present with signs of raised intracranial pressure—headache, nausea, papilledema, and VI nerve paresis. May also have vertigo, nystagmus, and ataxia
2. Syrinx
   a. May be located in the spinal cord or brainstem
   b. Symptoms include weakness and atrophy of the hands and arms, pain, and nystagmus
3. Endolymphatic sac tumors
   a. Have been found to have the same genetic defects as other VHL tumors
   b. Patients present with hearing loss, tinnitus, vertigo, and facial weakness

G. Visceral lesions

1. Renal cell carcinoma
2. Pheochromocytoma
3. Benign cysts of the kidneys, pancreas, liver, and epididymis
4. Polycythemia: the central nervous system hemangioblastoma produces erythropoietin

H. Diagnostic criteria: patients must have one manifestation of the syndrome and a family member with a CNS hemangioblastoma

VII. Sturge-Weber syndrome (SWS)

A. Also known as encephalotrigeminal angiomatosis

B. Rare syndrome

C. Hereditary pattern is unknown. Patients with SWS have normal karyotypes

D. Facial lesion—facial angioma
　1. This lesion is also referred to as a port-wine stain or a nevus flammeus
　2. Present at birth
　3. The reddish-purple lesion is usually unilateral and follows cutaneous distribution of V^1 and V^2. V^3 is less often affected. One, two, or all three dermatomes may be involved simultaneously
　4. Facial angiomas can be bilateral. Some patients have extensive lesions that involve the trunk and limbs
　5. Port-wine stain is associated with hemihypertrophy of the face

E. Ocular lesions
　1. Glaucoma is seen in 60% of patients with SWS. Sixty percent of patients will develop glaucoma prior to age 2
　　a. Glaucoma is usually ipsilateral to the facial angioma
　　b. More common in patients with facial angiomas involving the upper eyelid
　　c. Glaucoma is believed to be secondary to an anterior chamber angle anomaly and/or elevated episcleral venous pressure
　　d. Glaucoma difficult to control
　2. Choroidal hemangioma
　　a. Seen in 40% of patients with SWS
　　b. Ipsilateral to the facial angioma
　　c. Two types
　　　i. Diffuse choroidal angioma is the most common—"tomato ketchup fundus"
　　　ii. Localized angiomas
　　d. Can cause hyperopia and retinal degeneration
　3. Heterochromia iridis—the iris ipsilateral to the facial angioma may be deeply pigmented
　4. Angiomas of the conjunctiva and sclera

F. Central nervous system lesion—leptomeningeal hemangioma
　1. The angioma is located between the pia and arachnoid
　2. Ipsilateral to the facial angioma; 15% of lesions are bilateral
　3. Most often located over the parieto-occipital cortex
　4. Underlying cortex is maldeveloped and hypoplastic
　　a. Cortical veins are absent or nonfunctional
　　b. Calcium deposited within the blood vessels and superficial layers of the cortex. Produces "tram-track" appearance on cranial CT scanning
　5. Consequences of cortical and meningeal lesions
　　a. Seventy-five percent will have contralateral seizures
　　b. Fifty-five to 85% of patients will have some form of learning disability
　　c. Hemiplegia
　　d. Homonymous visual field defect

G. No visceral lesions

H. Diagnostic criteria—patients must have two of these criteria
1. Facial angioma with ipsilateral intracranial hemangioma
2. Ipsilateral choroidal hemangioma
3. Congenital glaucoma

VIII. Wyburn-Mason syndrome (WMS)

A. Also known as retinocephalic vascular malformation

B. Incidence and hereditary pattern unknown

C. Cutaneous lesions rare. Some patients have a facial angioma

D. Ocular lesions
1. Arteriovenous malformation (AVM) of the retina
   a. This lesion is also known as a racemose angioma
   b. It is unilateral and most often located in the posterior pole
   c. Visual acuity can range from 20/20 to NLP
2. Orbital AVM
3. Optic nerve AVM

E. Central nervous system lesion—AVM of the CNS
1. Ipsilateral to the retinal AVM
2. Fifty percent will be symptomatic

F. Visceral lesions—patients may have AVMs of the ipsilateral maxilla, pterygoid fossa, mandible, and spine

G. Diagnostic criteria—the classic WMS consists of an intracranial AVM and separate retinal AVM

IX. Ataxia-telangiectasia (A-T)

A. Also known as Louis-Bar syndrome

B. A-T occurs at a frequency of eight per million live births

C. Genetics
1. Inherited as an autosomal recessive trait
2. The A-T gene is on chromosome 11 (11q22-23)
3. The A-T gene encodes a protein called ATM, which is important for cell cycle control and DNA repair

D. Cutaneous lesion—telangiectasias of the skin
1. Occurs on exposed areas of skin—ears, nose, neck
2. Usually presents around age 4

E. Ocular lesions
1. Bilateral bulbar conjunctival telangiectasia
   a. Appears between the ages of 3 and 6
   b. Becomes more prominent with age
2. Ocular motility disturbances
   a. Patients first develop oculomotor apraxia
   b. Later, impairment of smooth pursuit
   c. Eventually, complete supranuclear ophthalmoplegia

F. Central nervous system lesion—atrophy of the cerebellum

1. Atrophy particularly prominent in the cerebellar cortex and vermis
2. Clinical consequences of cerebellar atrophy
   a. Cerebellar ataxia becomes evident when the patient begins to walk; progressive; patients are wheelchair bound by age 10
   b. Dysarthria
   c. Chorea
   d. Dystonia
   e. Regression of intellectual milestones

G. Visceral lesions
1. Respiratory infections are frequent
   a. Hypoplastic thymus
   b. Hypoplasia of tonsils, adenoids, and lymphoid tissue
   c. Deficiency of IgG2, IgG4, IgA, and IgE
2. Patients with A-T have poor auto-DNA repair after exposure to ultraviolet light and radiation. This leads to a 100-fold increased cancer rate. They often develop leukemia and lymphoma
3. Elevated α-fetoprotein level

H. Diagnostic criteria
1. Characteristic neurologic features:
   a. Gait ataxia in the first 2 or 3 years of life
   b. Ocular motor signs and dysarthria by early school years. Subsequent movement disorders, worsening limb ataxia, facial hypomimia, swallowing incoordination, and peripheral neuropathy
2. At least one of the following:
   a. Ocular telangiectasia
   b. Elevated serum α-fetoprotein level after 1 year of age
   c. Spontaneous or radiation-induced chromosomal breakage (colony survival DNA analysis)

X. Klippel-Trénaunay-Weber syndrome (KTWS)

A. KTWS is a sporadic disorder. Incidence and mode of inheritance is unknown

B. KTWS is characterized by the following triad:
1. Cutaneous vascular abnormalities
2. Varicosities
3. Bony and soft tissue hypertrophy

C. Most common site is leg, followed by arm, trunk, and rarely head and neck

D. Cutaneous lesion—port-wine stain
1. Present at birth
2. Found in 98% of patients with KTWS
3. Darkens and thickens with age

E. Ophthalmologic manifestations
1. Port-wine stain of the face
2. Orbital varix
3. Heterochromia irides

  4. Varicosities of the retina
  5. Choroidal angioma

F. Central nervous system lesions uncommon

G. Visceral lesions
  1. Varicose veins
    a. May be present at birth, but usually obvious during childhood
    b. Complications: lymphedema, stasis ulceration, pulmonary embolism
  2. Hypertrophy of bone and soft tissues
    a. Causes an increase in both length and girth of affected extremity
    b. Progressive during first several years of life
    c. Disproportionate enlargement of a single extremity can cause scoliosis and gait abnormalities

H. Diagnostic criteria—patient must have two of these criteria
  1. Cutaneous vascular abnormality
  2. Soft tissue and/or bony hypertrophy
  3. Varicose veins

BIBLIOGRAPHY

Chapters

Selhorst JB. Phacomatoses. In: Miller NR, Newman NJ, eds. *Walsh and Hoyt's Clinical Neuro-ophthalmology*. 5th ed. Vol 2. Baltimore, Md: Williams & Wilkins; 1998: 2647-2744.

Shields JA, Shields CA. Systemic hamartomases. In: Manis MJ, Macsai MS, Huntley AC, eds. *Eye and Skin Disease*. Philadelphia, Pa: Lippincott-Raven; 1998: chapter 45, 367-380.

Articles

Cabana MD, Crawford TO, Winkelstein JA, et al. Consequences of the delayed diagnosis of ataxia-telangiectasia. *Pediatrics*. 1998;102:98-100.

Destro M, D'Amico DJ, Gragoudas ES, et al. Retinal manifestations of neurofibromatosis: diagnosis and management. *Arch Ophthalmol*. 1991;109:662-666.

Evans DG. Neurofibromatosis type 2: genetic and clinical features. *ENT J*. 1999;78:97-100.

Filling-Katz MR, Choyke PL, Oldfield E, et al. Central nervous system involvement in von Hippel-Lindau disease. *Neurology*. 1991;41:41-46.

Jacob AG, Driscoll DJ, Shaughnessy WJ, et al. Klippel-Trénaunay syndrome: spectrum and management. *Mayo Clin Proc*. 1998;73:28-36.

Karnes PS. Neurofibromatosis: a common neurocutaneous disorder. *Mayo Clin Proc*. 1998;73:1071-1076.

Kaye LD, Rothner AD, Beauchamp GR, et al. Ocular findings associated with neurofibromatosis type II. *Ophthalmology*. 1999;99:1424-1429.

Lewis RF, Lederman HM, Crawford TO. Ocular motor abnormalities in ataxia-telangiectasia. *Ann Neurol*. 1999;46:287-295.

MacDonald IM, Bech-Hansen NT, Britton WA, et al. The phakomatoses: recent advances in genetics. *Can J Ophthalmol*. 1997;32:4-11.

Meine JG, Schwartz RA, Janniger CK. Klippel-Trénaunay-Weber syndrome. *Pediat Derm*. 1997;60:127-132.

Patel U, Gupta SC. Wyburn-Mason syndrome: a case report and review of the literature. *Neuroradiology*. 1990;31:544-546.

Weiner DM, Ewalt DH, Roach ES, Hensle TW. The tuberous sclerosis complex: a comprehensive review. *J Am Coll Surg*. 1998;187:548-561.

Chapter 20

Ancillary Clinical Procedures

Patrick S. O'Connor, MD

I.   **Superficial temporal artery biopsy**

A. The temporal artery is a terminal branch of the external carotid artery. Because of its ready accessibility and high frequency of involvement in giant cell arteritis, it is most often biopsied to establish the diagnosis

B. The artery lies in front of the ear over the zygomatic process of the temporal bone. It divides into a posterior parietal branch and anterior frontal branch (Figure 20-1A). The frontal branch lies above the temporalis fascia and follows a tortuous course across the forehead to an anastomosis with the supraorbital and supratrochlear branches of the ophthalmic artery

C. The frontal branch is usually chosen for biopsy. The artery is classically described as being nodular and tender when involved. However, the vessel may feel and look normal, yet prove abnormal on histologic examination

D. After the frontal branch is identified, the area should be prepared by shaving the overlying skin

E. The shaved area is scrubbed with Betadine solution for 5 minutes with 4 x 4's. The area is then dried and a sterile plastic eye drape is applied to the biopsy area

F. The vessel is carefully palpated and its course marked for 4 to 5 cm

G. Plain 2% xylocaine is used for local infiltration. Epinephrine should be avoided because of its vasospastic potential. Five to 10 cc should be injected 1 cm to either side of the artery and parallel to, but not directly over, the artery itself

H. The skin incision is made with a No. 15 Bard Parker blade (Becton Dickinson, Franklin Lakes, NJ) directly along the skin mark. Traction at each end of the incision site is used when making the full-thickness incision through the skin. 4 x 4's can then be used at the incision edges to control bleeding. Rarely is cautery or ligature needed

I. Subcutaneous blunt dissection is done using a hemostat or small blunt-nosed scissors. Dissection with sharp instruments is never performed. The frontal branch is identified above the temporalis fascia (Figure 20-1B)

J. If pulsations were obtained at the beginning of the procedure, the dissection bed is repeatedly palpated to identify the course of the artery

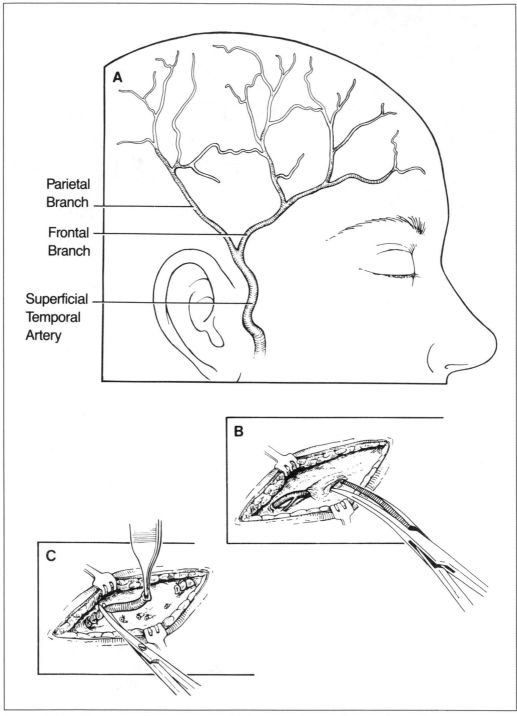

Figure 20-1. Steps in performing a superficial temporal artery biopsy. A. Localization. B. Blunt dissection. C. Removal of biopsy specimen.

K. If the pulse disappears, several drops of proparacaine can be instilled on the wound, reducing vasospasm

L. Two 4-0 black silk sutures are passed below the artery, one proximally and one distally to permit manipulation without the use of instruments that could cause crush artifact. At least 3 cm of artery should be isolated and freed from surrounding tissue. Branches of the artery are ligated with 4-0 chromic sutures. The artery is ligated as far proximally and distally as possible. Three square knots should be placed with the silk sutures and the ends not cut too closely. Some prefer a double ligature proximally and distally (Figure 20-1C)

M. Once bleeding is controlled, the wound is closed with 6-0 nylon sutures. A pressure dressing is applied for 24 hours

N. The most common late complication is hemorrhage. There is one case report of a patient with asymptomatic internal carotid occlusion who suffered a stroke during biopsy of the ipsilateral temporal artery because of interruption of collateral flow. It may be prudent to compress the vessel for several minutes to ensure that critical collateral flow will not be compromised if it is removed

O. Skin sutures are removed in 5 days

II. **The Tensilon test**

A. Tensilon (edrophonium hydrochloride) is supplied in a single dose, 10 mg/1 mL breakneck vial

B. A definite endpoint must be selected. If the patient has no findings at the time of examination, testing should be postponed. If ptosis is present, it should be documented photographically before and after injection

C. If diplopia is present careful measurement of the deviation should be carried out before, immediately after, and 3 to 4 minutes following injection. Three types of responses may occur in myasthenic patients. Type 1 responses occur only in myasthenics while type 2 and 3 responses may be seen in nonmyasthenic ophthalmoplegia:
   1. An improvement in alignment (large tropia becomes smaller)
   2. A worsening of alignment (a small tropia becomes a large tropia)
   3. A reversal of alignment (a left hypertropia becomes a right hypertropia)

D. Procedure in adults:
   1. Tensilon should be drawn up in a 1 cc tuberculin syringe
   2. 0.4 mg of injectable atropine should also be drawn up in another 1 cc tuberculin syringe
   3. A 10 cc syringe is filled with injectable saline
   4. A scalp vein needle is placed in a dorsal arm or hand vein
   5. 1 mL of saline solution is injected and the patient observed for 1 minute
   6. 0.2 mL of Tensilon is injected and the tubing flushed with 1 mL of saline, then observed for 1 minute
   7. If no response, a bolus of 0.8 mL of Tensilon is injected and the tubing flushed with another 1 mL of saline; atropine is then connected to the tubing
   8. Atropine (0.4 mg intramuscularly [IM]) may be used to pretreat all patients 15 minutes before Tensilon testing, or used intravenously only to avoid undesirable cholinergic side effects (eg, bradycardia, angina, bronchospasm)

E. In children and uncooperative adults, 0.4 mg of atropine is given intramuscularly 15 minutes prior to the injection of neostigmine (Prostigmin) and the dose calculated as follows: weight (kg)/70 (kg) times 1.5 mg = dose. Patient is reexamined 30 to 45 minutes after injection

III. **Forced duction testing (Figure 20-2)**

A. In patients with acquired diplopia and an incomitant deviation, forced duction testing can eliminate the need for extensive neurologic investigation if restriction is found. Remember, many patients with thyroid myopathy have only subtle or no other signs of classic thyroid eye disease

B. Three drops of topical proparacaine solution are instilled in the inferior cul-de-sac of each eye. During this time, a cotton-tipped applicator is soaked with similar solution

C. The patient is asked to look in the direction of gaze limitation. The cotton-tipped applicator is placed on the conjunctiva anterior to the presumed restricted muscle

D. The conjunctiva is grasped with toothed forceps and the globe passively rotated in the direction of the limited duction

E. The same procedure is carried out in the fellow eye and the relative limitation compared. In subtle cases, repeated comparisons between the two eyes may be necessary

F. At times with attempted forced ductions, the globe is displaced backward into the orbit. This phenomenon must be observed, or the examiner may believe the eye moves more easily than it actually does

G. Occasionally, patients are not able to cooperate for forced duction testing. In these cases, measurement of the intraocular pressure in the primary position and again with the eyes moved into the direction of limited gaze is compared. A pressure rise of greater than 4 mm in moving from one gaze position to another is felt to be diagnostic of a restrictive process

IV. **Confrontation visual fields**

A. Many significant neurologic field defects can be found with simple confrontation techniques

B. The best technique of finger-counting fields evaluates both sides of the vertical meridian with care taken not to move the fingers in various quadrants since many patients with a damaged occipital lobe can still appreciate motion in the blind field (Riddoch phenomenon)

C. Procedure (Figure 20-3):

1. One eye of the patient is occluded

2. The patient is then asked to look at the examiner's nose while maintaining steady fixation. The test distance should be approximately 1 m between patient and examiner

3. Finger counting is then carried out in the four quadrants: superior temporal, inferior temporal, inferior nasal, and superior nasal. Between one and five fingers is presented and the number varied. The fingers are presented in a static fashion 20 degrees and 30 degrees from fixation

4. Double simultaneous stimulation (Oppenheim's test). The same number of fingers are simultaneously presented on each side of the vertical meridian with careful monitoring of the patient's fixation. Parietal lobe lesions can result in visual field inattention to simultaneous targets even when individually presented targets can be identified

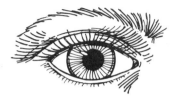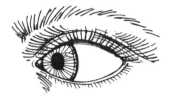

A. ABDUCTION DEFECT RIGHT EYE

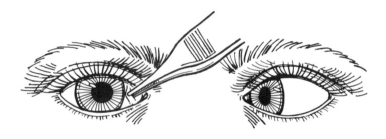

B. POSITIVE FORCED DUCTION TEST
Resistance to abduction of right eye

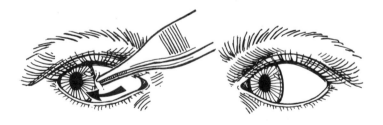

C. NEGATIVE FORCED DUCTION TEST
No resistance to abduction of right eye

Figure 20-2. Forced duction testing.

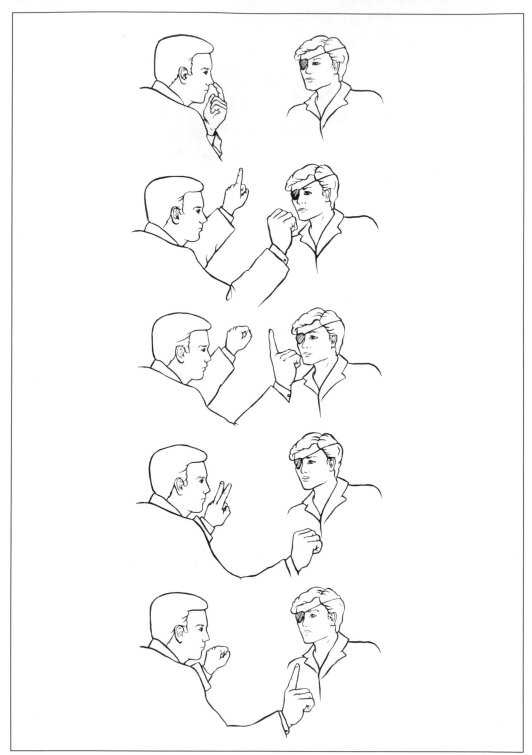

Figure 20-3. Confrontation visual field technique.

5. Hemifield comparison. Again with controlled fixation, both hands are held on either side of the vertical meridian and the patient is asked to compare their appearance (ie, one "clearer" or "darker" than the other). The patient is always asked to point to the abnormal hand to reduce confusion. If, for example, the hand in the patient's temporal field appears dimmer, then both hands are again presented in the temporal field above and below the horizontal, and the patient is asked to identify the clearer of the two, allowing definition of whether the defect is denser above or below

6. The same procedure is carried out in the other eye

D. Finger-counting fields should be performed as part of every routine examination not just in patients suspected of having neurologic disease

E. A great deal of information can also be gained from subjective visual fields in which the patient covers one eye and focuses on the center of the examiner's face, usually the nose. The patient is then asked if he or she can see both ears simultaneously, the head, the chin, the examiner's shoulder, tie, etc. Frequently, scotomas not easily identified on perimetry are recognized as a central dimming by the patient when viewing the examiner's face. The same is also true for early inferior altitudinal defects that may be subtle on perimetry but easily identified by the patient on subjective examination

V.   Optic nerve sheath decompression (Figure 20-4)

A. The orbital optic nerve can be approached surgically either medially or laterally

B. The medial approach is preferred, since it is technically easier and quicker, and avoids removal of the lateral bony orbital wall

C. A speculum is used to open the lids, and a lateral canthotomy is performed

D. A medial conjunctival peritomy is made, the medial rectus muscle is isolated on a muscle hook, a double-armed 6-0 coated Vicryl suture (Ethicon J-570, Somerville, NJ) is passed though the muscle close to its insertion, and the muscle is disinserted from the globe

E. Another double-armed 6-0 Vicryl suture (J-556) is woven through the stump of the medial rectus insertion, and this suture is used to pull the eye into an abducted position (see Figure 20-4A)

F. Single-armed 5-0 Dacron sutures (Davis & Geck 2919-23, Manati, Puerto Rico) are passed through partial-thickness sclera in the superonasal and inferonasal quadrants (see Figure 20-4A)

G. The two Dacron sutures are pulled firmly to position the eye in full abduction (see Figure 20-4A)

H. A malleable orbital retractor is placed between the disinserted medial rectus muscle and the globe to expose the optic nerve immediately behind the globe

I. Cotton-tipped applicators and cottonoids are used to retract orbital fat

J. The intrascleral course of the long posterior ciliary artery leads directly to the optic nerve

K. Once exposed, an avascular segment of the nerve sheath is selected for fenestration

L. Incision of the sheath is made with a sharp blade (MVR Untitome 5560, Beaver Surgical, Waltham, Mass) and extended approximately 5 mm (Figure 20-4B)

M.A gush of cerebrospinal fluid is often seen with the initial incision

N. Adhesions between the meninges and optic nerve are broken by passing a tenotomy or nerve hook into the fenestration (Figure 20-4C)

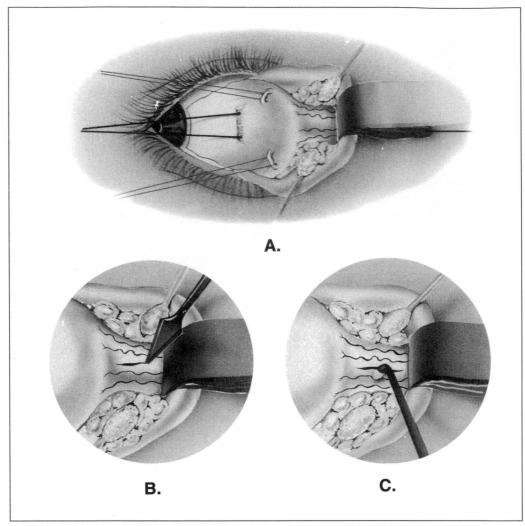

A.

B.   **C.**

Figure 20-4. Medial approach for optic nerve sheath decompression (see text for details).

O. Two to four fenestrations are made routinely, with lysis of the underlying adhesions

P. Meticulous attention to hemostasis is required

Q. The traction sutures are removed and the medial rectus is reattached at its original insertion

R. The medial conjunctival incision is closed with an absorbable suture

BIBLIOGRAPHY

Chapters

Anderson DR. *Perimetry: With and Without Automation.* 2nd ed. St. Louis, Mo: CV Mosby; 1987: 228-249.

Burde RM, Savino PJ, Trobe JD. *Clinical Decisions in Neuro-ophthalmology.* St. Louis, Mo: CV Mosby; 1992: 242-243.

Articles

Brennan J, McCrary JA. Diagnosis of superficial temporal arteritis. *Ann Ophthalmol.* 1975;7:1125-1129.

Plotnik JL, Kosmorsky GS. Operative complications of optic nerve sheath decompression. *Ophthalmology.* 1993;100:683-690.

Sergott RC. Optic nerve sheath decompression. *Intl Ophthalmol Clin.* 1991;31:71-81.

Shahinfar S, Johnson LN, Madsen RW. Confrontation visual field loss as a function of decibel sensitivity loss on automatic static perimetry. *Ophthalmology.* 1995;102:872-877.

Trobe JD, Acosta PC, Krischer JP, et al. Confrontation visual field techniques in the detection of anterior visual pathway lesions. *Ann Neurol.* 1981;10:28-34.

Tse DT, Nerad JA, Anderson RL, et al. Optic nerve sheath fenestration in pseudotumor cerebri. *Arch Ophthalmol.* 1988;106:1458-1462.

Index